J. Grifka D.J. Ogilvie-Harris (Eds.) · Osteoarthritis

Springer
Berlin
Heidelberg
New York
Barcelona
Hong Kong
London
Milan
Paris
Singapore
Tokyo

J. GRIFKA D.J. OGILVIE-HARRIS
Editors

Osteoarthritis

Fundamentals and Strategies for Joint-Preserving Treatment

With 102 Figures, 46 in Colour, and 36 Tables

Springer

Joachim Grifka, MD
Professor of Orthopaedic Surgery
Department of Orthopaedics, St. Josef-Hospital
Ruhr-University Bochum
Gudrunstrasse 56, 44791 Bochum, Germany

Darrell J. Ogilvie-Harris, MD
Professor of Orthopaedic Surgery
University of Toronto and the Toronto Hospital
Edith Cavell Wing 1-032
399 Bathurst Street, Toronto M5T 2S8, Canada

ISBN 978-3-642-87754-4

Cataloging-in-Publication Data applied for.
Die Deutsche Bibliothek – CIP-Einheitsaufnahme
Osteoarthritis: fundamentals and strategies for joint preserving treatment; with 36 tables/ J. Grifka; D.J. Ogilvie-Harris (ed.). – Berlin; Heidelberg; New York; Barcelona; Hong Kong; London; Milan; Paris; Singapore; Tokyo: Springer, 2000
ISBN 978-3-642-87754-4 ISBN 978-3-642-87752-0 (eBook)
DOI 10.1007/978-3-642-87752-0

Production: PRO EDIT GmbH, Heidelberg, Germany
Cover design: design & production, Heidelberg, Germany
Typesetting: K+V Fotosatz GmbH, Beerfelden, Germany

Printed on acid-free paper SPIN 10725937 24/3135Di 5 4 3 2 1 0

Preface

Osteoarthritis is one of the biggest challenges in orthopaedics today. Knee joint surgery has gone through a revolution during the last two decades. In the 1980s arthroscopy found a wide-spread application, due to developments in technology, i.e. optical systems and miniaturized instruments. In the 1990s we experienced a significant improvement in knee endoprothetics with functionally optimized designs to avoid major stress and to support correct load distribution. Nevertheless, joint replacement means a surrender. It marks the limits of our capability to keep the joint itself in physiological function. Moreover, our possibilities for treating cartilage destruction by common arthroscopic techniques are limited to debridement and abrasion arthroplasty, which is controversial because of postoperative problems and fibrocartilage substitute tissue. For years arthroscopy has seemed to remain at a plateau.

Big expectations had been placed on laser cartilage smoothing, but laser treatment has not yielded convincing results in follow-ups over the last five years; new laser techniques are yet to be seen.

On the other hand an increasing number of people are reaching old age, causing a higher percentage of our population to suffer from osteoarthritis with typical symptoms such as swelling, reduced mobility and restricted fitness for everyday life. Moreover, we are facing specific problems of osteoarthritis in young and middle-aged people due to cartilage destruction.

Due to these different circumstances the authors felt that there was a need to present today's knowledge of the pathogenesis and biomechanics of osteoarthritis, the different operative techniques for joint preservation and conservative treatment. We are happy that we can present a collection of contributions from leading experts working in the different fields for many years. As new techniques for cartilage restoration, such as autologous chondrocyte transplantation or bone cartilage transposition are the focus of clinical and scientific analyses we also gave room to present these.

We like to thank all the contributors for sharing their experience with us, giving us an overview of the different aspects of joint-preserving treatment. We are optimistic that this synopsis will enhance our understanding of present concepts, initiate further discussion, help us to assess our own points of view and hopefully to develop ideas for further improvement.

For considerable financial support for this project we should like to thank the Ministry of Schools and Education, Sciences and Research of Nordrhein-Westfalen.

Autumn 1999

JOACHIM GRIFKA
DARRELL J. OGILVIE-HARRIS

Contents

Contributors

JENS AGNESKIRCHER, MD
Department of Orthopaedic Sports Medicine
Technical University of Munich
Connollystrasse 32
80809 München, Germany

MATS BRITTBERG, MD, PhD, SOBE
Cartilage Research Unit, Department of Orthopaedics
Kungsbacka Hospital
S-43440 Kungsbacka, Sweden

ELIANE BROLL-ZEITVOGEL, MD
Parkklinik Bad Rothenfelde, Parkstrasse 12–14
49214 Bad Rothenfelde, Germany

JÜRGEN BRUNS, MD
Professor of Orthopaedic Surgery
Department of Orthopaedic Surgery, University of Hamburg
Martinistrasse 52
20246 Hamburg, Germany

ANDREAS BURKART, MD
Department of Orthopaedic Sports Medicine
Technical University of Munich
Connollystrasse 32
80809 München, Germany

CHONG-HYUK CHOI, MD
Assistant Professor,
Department of Orthopaedic Surgery
Yonsie University, College of Medicine
Seoul, Korea

KLAUS K. FÖRSTER, PhD
Igelweg 3
51766 Engelskirchen, Germany

JOACHIM GRIFKA, MD
Professor of Orthopaedic Surgery
Department of Orthopaedics, St. Josef-Hospital
Ruhr-University Bochum, Gudrunstrasse 56
44791 Bochum, Germany

MARKUS HEIN, MD
Department of Orthopaedics, Martin-Luther-University
Halle-Wittenberg, Magdeburger Strasse 22
06097 Halle (Saale), Germany

ANDREAS IMHOFF, MD
Professor of Orthopaedic Surgery
Director Department of Orthopaedic Sports Medicine
Technical University of Munich, Connollystrasse 32
80809 München, Germany

KEITA ITO, MD, ScD
Group Head, Cartilage Biomechanics, AO ASIF Research Institute
Clavadelerstrasse
7270 Davos Platz, Switzerland

THOMAS KALTEIS, MD
Department for Surgery, Klinikum Innenstadt
Ludwig-Maximilians-University Munich, Pettenkoferstrasse 8
80336 München, Germany

JOHANN KIRMAIR, MD
Vor den Eichen 1
32756 Detmold, Germany

STEFAN KLUG, MD
Department of Orthopaedic Rheumatology
Friedrich-Alexander-University Erlangen-Nürnberg
Waldkrankenhaus St. Marien, Rathsberger Strasse 57
91054 Erlangen, Germany

DJORDJE LAZOVIC, MD
Associate Professor, Orthopaedic Department
Medizinische Hochschule Hannover, Heimchenstrasse 1–7
30625 Hannover, Germany

ARNDT-MATTHIAS MÜLLER, MD
Department of Orthopaedics, Ruhr-University Bochum
St. Josef-Hospital, Gudrunstrasse 56
44791 Bochum, Germany

WINFRIED MOHR, MD
Professor of Pathology, Department of Pathology
University of Ulm, Albert-Einstein-Allee 11
89081 Ulm, Germany

STEFAN NEHRER, MD
Associate Professor, Department of Orthopaedic Surgery
University of Vienna, Währinger Gürtel 18
1090 Wien, Austria

DARRELL J. OGILVIE-HARRIS, MD
Professor of Orthopaedic Surgery
University of Toronto and the Toronto Hospital
Edith Cavell Wing 1-032, 399 Bathurst Street
Toronto M5T 2S8, Canada

GEORG OETTL, MD
Department of Orthopaedic Sports Medicine
Technical University of Munich, Connollystrasse 32
80809 München, Germany

WOLFGANG PLITZ, MD, PhD, Professor Dr.-Ing.
University Clinic of Orthopaedic Surgery
Klinikum Großhadern, Marchionistrasse 15
81377 München, Germany

HEIKO REICHEL, MD
Associate Professor of Orthopaedic Surgery
Department of Orthopaedics, Martin Luther-University
Halle-Wittenberg, Magdeburger Strasse 22
06097 Halle (Saale), Germany

OLIVER SANGHA, MD, MPH, MSc
Bavarian Public Health Research Center
Ludwig-Maximilians-University, Tegernseer Landstrasse 243
81549 München, Germany

PHILIP SCHÖTTLE, MD
Department of Orthopaedic Sports Medicine
Technical University of Munich
Connollystrasse 32
80809 München, Germany

WOLFGANG SCHULTZ, MD
Associate Professor of Orthopaedic Surgery
Department of Orthopaedics
Georg August-University Göttingen, Robert-Koch-Strasse 40
37075 Göttingen, Germany

MYRON SPECTOR, PhD
Department of Orthopaedic Surgery
Brigham and Women's Hospital, Harvard Medical School
Boston, MA, USA

JÜRGEN STEINMEYER, PhD
Department of Orthopaedics, Justus-Liebig-University Giessen
Paul Meimberg Strasse 3
35385 Giessen, Germany

SLOBADAN TEPIC, ScD
Rigistrasse 27B
8006 Zürich, Switzerland

JOACHIM TYWS, MD
Department of Orthopaedics, Ruhr-University Bochum
St. Josef-Hospital, Gudrunstrasse 56
44971 Bochum, Germany

GERD WESELOH, MD
Professor of Orthopaedic Surgery
Department of Orthopaedic Rheumatology
Friedrich-Alexander-University Erlangen-Nürnberg
Waldkrankenhaus St. Marien, Rathsberger Strasse 57
91054 Erlangen, Germany

MANFRED WILDNER, MD, MPH
Bavarian Public Health Research Center
Ludwig-Maximilians-University, Tegernseer Landstrasse 243
81549 München, Germany

DIRK WINDEMUTH, MPH, Dr. phil.
Berufsgenossenschaftliches Institut für Arbeit und Gesundheit
Alte Heerstr. 111
53757 St. Augustin

Epidemiologic and Economic Aspects of Osteoarthrosis

M. Wildner and O. Sangha

Epidemiologic Aspects

Introduction and Definitions

Osteoarthrosis (OA), i.e. degenerative joint disease, is the most common form of joint affection in humans and is responsible for a large proportion of morbidity in populations. It is of enormous economic importance in developed countries.

Research in OA has been complicated through a variable use of definitions, mainly centered around the question whether radiological criteria, clinical criteria, or a combination of both are used.

Although various definitions of OA have been proposed, it was not until 1986 that an explicit *standard definition for OA* was developed by the Subcommittee on OA of the American College of Rheumatology Diagnostic and Therapeutic Criteria Committee: "A heterogeneous group of conditions that lead to joint symptoms and signs which are associated with defective integrity of articular cartilage, in addition to related changes in the underlying bone at the joint margins" (Altman et al. 1986; Altman 1991).

The diagnosis of OA in epidemiological studies, as well as in clinical medicine, can be made by *history taking* (e.g. structured questionnaire), by *physical examination* (e.g. in a study center or by field investigation) or by *special technical examinations* (e.g. X-rays or laboratory exams). Traditionally, diagnosis of OA in epidemiological studies has relied on radiological examinations, with reference to the typical joint and bone characteristics described in the *Atlas of Standard Radiographs* (University of Manchester 1973). Such characteristics relate to: (a) osteophyte formation, (b) periarticular ossicles, (c) narrowing of joint space and sclerosis, (d) cysts and (e) deformity. Assessment of these changes are expressed on an ordinary severity scale with the expression 0 (normal), 1 (doubtful), 2 (minimal), 3 (moderate) and 4 (severe).

Furthermore, the cited Committee of the American College of Rheumatology proposed a *classification of subsets of osteoarthrosis* (Table 1).

In addition to diagnostic definitions, descriptive measures of disease frequency should be of explicit nature. Is the investigation directed to-

Table 1. Classification of OA (Subcommittee on OA of the American College of Rheumatology Diagnostic and Therapeutic Criteria Committee)

I	Idiopathic	
	A	Localized (1 = hands, 2 = feet, 3 = hip, 4 = knee, 5 = spine, 6 = other single sites)
	B	Generalized
II	Secondary	
	A	Post-traumatic
	B	Congenital or development disease (1 = localized, 2 = generalized)
	C	Calcium deposition disease
	D	Other bone and joint disorders
	E	Other diseases

Table 2. Epidemiologic concepts for disease frequency: prevalence and incidence

Prevalence	Number of existing cases in a population [a]
Incidence	Number of new cases in a population [b]

[a] Total population, at a point in time or over a period of time.
[b] Study population, which does *not* have the disease at the beginning. May be replaced by *person time*, i.e. the product of individuals and their contributing observed time in the study.

wards the risk estimates of *getting* OA *(incidence)*, or the risk of *having* OA (*prevalence*)? Table 2 differentiates between these two distinct concepts.

Moreover, it is necessary to define the *time frame* of an investigation in OA patients. Does "having OA" mean that osteoarthrotic symptoms or signs need to be present right at the moment the question is posed (*point prevalence*)? Does it refer to the past, e.g. 1 or 3 months (*period prevalence*)? Or does it refer to one's lifetime up to now?

Disease Frequency

Compared to other countries, e.g. the United States or the United Kingdom, there are basically no epidemiological data about large-scale radiographic surveys in Germany. Questionnaire-based national health surveys are of limited use because the diagnosis of OA requires advanced examinations, e.g. radiological methods. However, questionnaire-derived data can be supplemented with other information sources to derive an estimate of OA prevalence in Germany. About 5 million people (6% of the population), suffer from OA at any time (point prevalence), without consideration of back pain, and the prevalence over a period of months is estimated at 15 million. This difference in the prevalence figures is due to remission of symptoms and relatively pain-free intervals in the course of this chronic disease.

In principle, every joint can be affected by OA, with large joints of the lower extremity and the spine being predominantly involved. Table 3 gives estimations for the prevalence of OA in Germany.

This estimation is potentially not satisfactory, not only because the data have been derived indirectly, but also because it aggregates OA of various types and different origin (see Table 1). Several international studies have made a population-based assessment using X-ray examination of several joints. Table 4 gives an example for three common localizations of OA.

Risk Factors

Epidemiological studies allow the identification of risk factors as long as biologic plausibility is given and if other competing explanations or factors of known influence are controlled for. Examples for such "other fac-

Table 3. Estimated point prevalence (as percentage) of arthropathies and osteoarthrosis in Germany: stratified by age and sex

Arthropathies			Osteoarthrosis	
Age (years)	Men	Women	Men	Women
25–29	3.3	3.3	0.4	0.4
30–39	4.6	5.3	0.8	0.9
40–49	7.7	12.5	2.2	3.6
50–59	18.5	25.5	8.1	10.7
60–69	23.7	27.7	13.4	16.1
Total	11.8	15.4	5.0	6.5

Source: DHP-Survey 1990–1991, own estimates of point prevalence.

Table 4. Point prevalence of osteoarthrosis by radiological criteria in The Netherlands for the distal interphalangeal joints of the hand (DIP-joint), the knee and the hip

	DIP-joint		Knee (right)		Hip (right)	
Age (years)	Men	Women	Men	Women	Men	Women
25–34	1.2	0.4	–	–	–	–
35–44	5.5	6.6	–	–	–	–
45–54	18.7	30.6	9.3	14.2	2.5	2.3
55–64	44.3	61.5	16.8	18.6	7.8	3.1
65–74	54.7	75.5	20.8	26.1	8.5	12.5

The figures in the table represent the percentage of affected persons in the study population. Source: Zoertermeer Community Survey (Van Sasse et al. 1989).

tors" (confounders) are age and sex, which clearly have a strong independent effect on the risk of developing OA and this may be associated with "candidate" risk factors such as being overweight or assumed protective factors such as osteoporosis. A distinction may also be made between *modifiable* risk factors, such as obesity, and *not modifiable* risk factors such as age or gender. If biologic plausibility of an identified factor is uncertain, it is preferable to use the term *risk predictor* until a causal relationship has been established.

Epidemiologic evidence for risk factors is of an indirect nature, based on statistical association excluding alternative explanations, and needs confirmation by other studies. Therefore, risk factors for OA should be divided into three groups based on the strength of the evidence: risk factors with widespread consensus, probable risk factors, and controversial risk factors. An overview of the current discussion about risk factors in OA is shown in Table 5.

The concept of a causal chain, i.e. risk factors with a varying causal "distance" to the disease, that start a sequence of (modifiable) events, and the concept of sufficient, necessary and partial causes as parts of more complex causal relationships are worthwhile of being considered briefly. One example would be the development of OA following a slight post-traumatic joint incongruency together with habitual joint instability and increasing weight due to limited activity – clearly a multicausal process with various risk factors interacting.

Further discussion of risk factors and estimations on the prevalence or incidence of OA changes for selected joints can be found in the epidemiological literature (Silman and Hochberg 1993; Hamermann 1997; Oliveria 1996). From an international perspective, age- and gender-specific rates for OA of the hip are highest in economically developed countries and low in developing countries (Murray and Lopez 1996a; Murray and Lopez 1996b). Possible explanations are body weight and height, genetic influences, socio-cultural influences including nutrition or sitting habits. This

Table 5. Risk factors for osteoarthrosis by degree of evidence

Consensus	Probable	Controversial
Age	Instability	Hysterectomy
Female sex	Overuse	Hyperuricemia
Obesity	Hereditary factors	Running
Joint disorder		Hormone replacement (female sex hormones)
Inflammatory arthritis		
Chondrocalcinosis		
Trauma		
Repetitive occupational trauma		

does not apply to OA of the knee joint, where prevalence rates are comparable across countries.

Economic Aspects

Costs of Illness

Economic evaluation is the *comparative analysis of alternative courses of action in terms of both their costs and their consequences* (Drummond et al. 1987). The most straightforward approach to quantify the economic consequences of OA is the calculation of *cost-of-illness (COI)*, which is generally categorised into *direct* medical costs (*spent resources*), such as hospital treatment, ambulatory care, medication or rehabilitation, and *indirect* macroeconomic costs (*lost resources*), including days off work, sickness pay, invalidity or premature mortality.

In Germany, direct medical costs for musculoskeletal diseases are estimated as high as 13.7 billion DM (7.7 billion US$) in 1990 (Henke et al. 1986; Henke et al. 1996, personal communication). About 100000 arthroscopies with cartilage smoothing are done annually in the ambulatory care sector, and there are about 140000 OA-related surgical procedures in hospitals with an average length of stay of 20 days. Costs for hospital treatment are averaged at 400 DM (220 US$) per day for an acute care setting and 240 DM (130 US$) in a rehabilitation facility. Hospital remuneration for a total hip replacement is currently 18600 DM (10000 US$) all inclusive (diagnosis-related group), 22600 DM (12500 US$) for a total knee replacement, and 5850 DM (3250 US$) for a hallux valgus arthroplasty. In the acute care and rehabilitation clinics combined 4.3 million hospital days are attributable to OA. Direct costs for OA are estimated at 6.3 billion DM (3.5 billion US$) in 1993 both in the hospital and in the ambulatory care sector, annual costs per case are currently estimated at 415 DM (230 US$) (Table 6).

Table 6. Cost-of-illness (COI) estimates for direct medical costs of osteoarthrosis in Germany in the mid-1990s

4.3 Million hospital days	1.5%	=2.0 Billion DM	1.1 Billion US$
Out-patient care	1.5%	>1.1 Billion DM [a]	>0.6 Billion US$
Medication/appliances		=1.8 Billion DM	1.0 Billion US$
Social/professional rehabilitation		=1.0 Billion DM	0.5 Billion US$
Long-term care		=0.4 Billion DM	0.2 Billion US$
Direct costs		>6.3 Billion DM [a]	3.5 Billion US$
Annual costs per case		>415 DM [a]	>230 US$

[a] Conservative estimate.

It is difficult to estimate indirect costs for OA. Death due to OA is a rare, although realistic event, mainly if adverse drug reactions (gastrointestinal bleeding) or postsurgical complications (thrombosis) occur, and may, age-dependently, result in loss of life years and loss of economic productivity.

In Germany, 6.6% of all early retirements, about 18000 cases in 1993, are related to OA. Accordingly, 6.7 million sickness days with an average duration of 39 days per incident are due to OA. Average monthly pension benefits are currently 1300 DM (720 US$), average benefit for each sickness day about 165 DM (91 US$). It has been suggested that indirect costs for arthropathies and osteopathies are about 1.6 times the direct medical costs (Brenner 1998), which would amount to 10 billion DM (5.5 billion US$) due to indirect costs. Consequently, total costs of illness for OA would add up to 16.3 billion (9.2 billion US$).

International comparisons of costs need expert knowledge because of differences in health care systems, cost accounting, and varying definitions and should be a reason to consult an experienced health economist (Liang et al. 1984; Sangha and Stucki 1997).

Advanced Economic Analyses

COI-analysis is only one approach out of multiple economic analyses that have emerged in the past 50 years in response to increasing financial constraints in the public and private health care sector. Table 7 gives an overview of advanced economic methods in health care.

Cost-minimization analysis is applied if the goal is to save costs for an established standard procedure without compromising quality, e.g. by lowering prices or changing processes. If several procedures are competing, claiming equal or superior effectiveness, then *cost-effectiveness* analyses give information on the costs involved with one predefined outcome, e.g. the avoidance of postoperative thromboembolic events. Particularly in chronic conditions or complex interventions with potentially multiple outcomes, cost-effectiveness analyses are of limited information, because the effect side is restricted to one outcome. An analysis of total joint replacement surgery that estimates cost-effectiveness of the intervention with respect to improvement of functional capacity would not be

Table 7. Advanced economic methods with application in the health care sector

Cost-minimization analysis (CMA)
Cost-effectiveness analysis (CEA)
Cost-utility analysis (CUA)
Cost-benefit analysis (CBA)

able to incorporate additional benefits (e.g. pain reduction) or potential adverse events (e.g. postoperative infections or thromboembolic events).

If procedures with multiple effects or different diseases are compared, *cost-benefit* analysis has been applied. This type of analysis considers both the costs (input) and potential effects of an intervention (output) in monetary terms, i.e. as future direct or indirect costs avoided by the implantation of an endoprosthesis, including the treatment costs for this intervention. Cost-benefit analysis has been criticized because certain outcomes (e.g. pain, a functional limitation or death) can hardly be expressed in monetary terms.

Cost–utility analyses differ from cost–benefit analysis as they aggregate outcomes not in monetary terms but in so-called *utilities*. A utility is an abstract construct that reflects an outcome in terms of a combination of morbidity and patient preferences, e.g. as a *quality adjusted life year (QUALY)* lost or gained by an intervention. A QUALY is the product of a life year times a "quality weight" assigned to it, ranging from 0 (worst case, near death) to 1 (perfect heath). Murray and Lopez (1996b) measure the "burden of disease" imposed to a population by *disability adjusted life years (DALY)* and estimate the proportion of DALYs attributable to OA in developed countries to be as high as that of dementia or lung cancer, larger than that of diabetes mellitus, and about one third of the burden of disease imposed by ischaemic heart disease.

Further economic analytical tools such as discounting, sensitivity analysis, marginal analysis, or decision analysis are beyond the scope of this introductory text.

Perspectives

Societies in developed countries are demographically "aging". The change from a population with a high birth rate and a high age-specific mortality, and consequently a moderate life expectancy at birth, to a population with a low birth rate and low age-specific mortality, and consequently a high life expectancy has been termed *demographic transition*. This transition can be visualized in population statistics and life tables by the change from a triangular population "pyramid" to a rectangular shape.

Demographic predictions suggest an increase of the total number of symptomatic cases by 15% up to the year 2010 in Germany, if age-specific incidence- and prevalence-rates are constant. Predictions for the USA are consistent with these figures, and the prevention and treatment of OA have been given high priority in preparing for the future of aging populations (Boult et al. 1996).

While a reduction of the prevalence of OA will reduce the number of functionally limited older persons, a reduction in the prevalence of coronary artery disease (CAD) or cancer most likely will not. This is a function of competing morbidity causing additional expenses if mortality is lowered, e.g. by a changing prevalence of CAD: people may live long enough to acquire another disabling condition. Allocation of society's limited resources will raise serious ethical questions, because interventions that are effective regarding mortality and morbidity will increasingly be evaluated regarding their economic efficiency (Wildner 1998). Effective treatment of OA has the potential to be cost-efficient both short- and long-term, but economic considerations should *not* be the only or major determinant for health care decisions.

References

Altman R, Asch E, Bloch D et al. (1986) Development of criteria for the classification and reporting of osteoarthritis: classification of osteoarthritis of the knee. Arthritis Rheum 29:1039–1049

Altman R (1991) Classification of disease: osteoarthritis. Semin Arthritis Rheum 20 [Suppl 2]:40–47

Brenner G (1998) Die volkswirtschaftliche Bedeutung der Arthrose. Orthopädie (Mitteilungen der DGOT) 2:15–24

Boult C, Altmann M, Gilbertson D, Yu C, Kane RL (1996) Decreasing disability in the 21st century: the future effects of controlling six fatal and nonfatal conditions. Am J Public Health 86:1388–1393

Drummond MF, Stoddart GL, Torrance GW (1987) Methods for the economic evaluation of health care programmes. Oxford Medical Publications, Oxford

Hamermann D (1997) Osteoarthritis. Johns Hopkins University Press, Baltimore, MD

Henke KD, Behrens C (1986) The economic cost of illness in the Federal Republic of Germany in the year 1980. Health Policy 6:119–143

Liang MH, Larson M, Thompson M (1984) Costs and outcomes in rheumatoid arthritis and osteoarthritis. Arthritis Rheum 27:522–529

Murray CJL, Lopez AD (1996a) Global health statistics. World Health Organization, Geneva

Murray CJL, Lopez AD (1996b) The global burden of disease. World Health Organization, Geneva

Oliveria SA, Felson DT, Klein RA (1996) Estrogen replacement therapy and the development of osteoarthritis. Epidemiology 7:415–419

Sangha O, Stucki G (1997) Economic impact of rheumatologic disorders. Curr Opin Rheumatol 9:102–105

Silman AJ, Hochberg MC (1993) Epidemiology of the rheumatic diseases. Oxford University Press, Oxford

University of Manchester, Department of Rheumatology and Medical Illustration (1973) Atlas of standard radiographs. Manchester University Press, Manchester

van Sasse JLCM, Vandenbroucke JB, van Romunde LKJ, Valkenburg HA (1989) Epidemiology of osteoarthritis: Zoertermeer survey. Comparison of radiologic osteoarthritis in a Dutch population with that in 10 other populations. Ann Rheum Dis 48:271–280

Wildner M (1998) Means and ends: cost effectiveness and overall costs. Am J Public Health 88:133

Clinical Picture of Osteoarthrosis

S. Klug and G. Weseloh

Introduction

In recent years, research into osteoarthrosis has provided numerous new facts that have deepened our knowledge and understanding of this disease and opened up new avenues of thought. Using biochemical and molecular-biological, pathomorphological, immunological, genetic and, in particular, clinical methods, we have succeeded in considerably expanding our knowledge of this disease. Nevertheless, many questions, in particular those concerned with aspects of treatment, still await definitive answers.

On the basis of the newly acquired data, osteoarthrosis is now being viewed, more than ever, as a multifactorial process. In the more common forms of osteoarthrosis affecting the large weight-bearing joints of the lower extremities, an imbalance between loading and loadability of the joints probably has an important role to play. Today, the conventional concept of wear and tear is no longer considered adequate to explain the osteoarthrotic process. It has also now been found that the usual classification of osteoarthrosis into primary and various secondary forms (Table 1) is often of only little practical use in the clinical setting, since, in many cases, a variety of interactions exist between the underlying causes. In the clinical area, a different consideration of the clinical picture may, therefore, provide useful information, in particular with regard to the treatment and prognosis of the illness. It is therefore of importance to be familiar with the various manifestations of osteoarthrosis and its specific risk factors, and then to apply this knowledge to treatment considerations.

In view of the wealth of new information, it is not possible to deal with all the unequivocal and current aspects of the clinical picture of osteoarthrosis in a short chapter, and we shall concentrate strictly on essentials.

The Osteoarthrotic Process

Buckwalter and Lane (1997) defined osteoarthrosis as a progressive loss of articular cartilage, which is associated with reparative reactions of the

Table 1. Classification of osteoarthrosis (Mankin 1986)

I. Primary (idiopathic)
   1. Localized
   2. Generalized (three or more areas)
   3. Erosive and inflammatory osteoarthritis
II. Secondary
   1. Congenital or developmental
      (a) Joint dysplasias
      (b) Joint and axis deviations
      (c) Slipped epiphysis
      (d) Bone dysplasias (epiphyseal dysplasia, spondylo-apophyseal dysplasia, osteochondrodystrophy)
      (e) Statically caused arthropathy (long leg arthropathy)
   2. Post-traumatic
      (a) Acute macrotrauma (incongruity, loss of stability, cartilage injury)
      (b) Chronic microtrauma (occupational, sports)
   3. Inflammatory joint diseases
      (a) Septic arthritis
      (b) Chronic gout arthritis
      (c) Rheumatoid diseases
   4. Metabolic
      (a) Chondrocalcinosis
      (b) Hemochromatosis (alkaptonuria)
      (c) Ochronosis
      (d) Wilson's disease
      (e) Paget's disease
   5. Endocrine
      (a) Diabetes mellitus
      (b) Acromegaly
      (c) Hypothyroidism
      (d) Hyperparathyroidism
      (e) Obesity
   6. Genetic
      (a) Type II collagen anomalies
      (b) Capsular collagen disturbances and hypermobility syndromes (e.g., Ehlers-Danlos syndrome)
   7. Neuropathic (Charcot joints, tabes dorsalis, syringomyelia, diabetes mellitus)
   8. Endemic
      (a) Kashin-Beck disease
      (b) Mseleni disease
   9. Miscellaneous
      (a) Frostbite
      (b) Caisson's disease
      (c) Hemoglobinopathies
   10. Various
      (a) Hemophilic arthropathy
      (b) Aseptic and avascular necrosis (Ahlbäck's disease, Legg-Calvé-Perthes disease, Osteochondrosis dissecans)

cartilage, remodeling processes and sclerosis of the subchondral bone, together with the formation of subchondral bone cysts and marginal osteophytes (Fig. 1). Involved in this process are numerous changes occurring at the molecular and cellular levels and leading to structural and functional loss affecting the articular cartilage, accompanied by secondary intra-articular processes (Boszotta et al. 1994).

Histological studies have shown that the destruction of articular cartilage in osteoarthrosis is initiated by fibrillation of the superficial zone. As the disease progresses, vertical and horizontal spreading of the defects with deep fissuring of the surface, separated fragments of cartilage within the articular cavity, and a decrease in cartilage thickness, progressing even to complete loss of cartilage, leaving denuded and eburnated subchondral bone (Fig. 2). Progressive joint destruction leads to incongruity of the articular surfaces, loss of ligament stability, axis deviations, and the formation of osteophytes. In later stages, these processes often lead to bizarre deformations of the joint (Fig. 3).

Clinical routine shows that osteoarthrosis does not necessarily lead to significant pain in those afflicted, and that in many cases, even quite advanced disease may be associated with surprisingly few symptoms.

Basically, the disease is a chronic process that develops over a period of years and decades. The clinical course, however, is usually not uniform, but often erratic. Initially, the clinical manifestation of the disease often remains non-progressive for years. During the further course of the illness, however, phases of mild symptoms may alternate with periods of

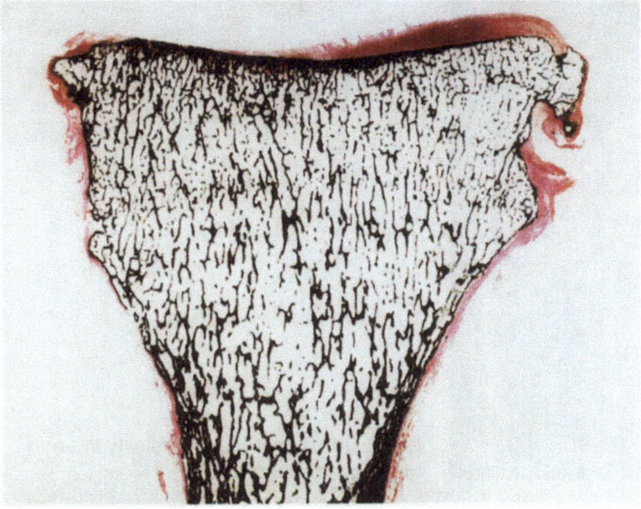

Fig. 1. Histological slide preparation of a human tibial head showing stage II–IV chondromalacia (safranin-O/von Kossa stain)

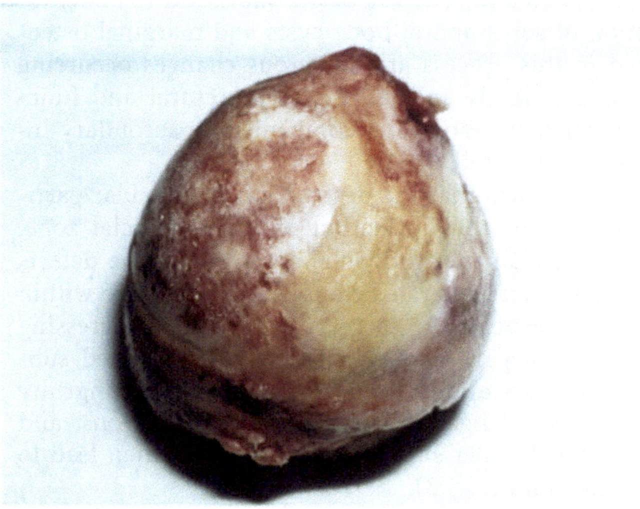

Fig. 2. Intra-operative femoral head specimen in advanced osteoarthrosis of the hip

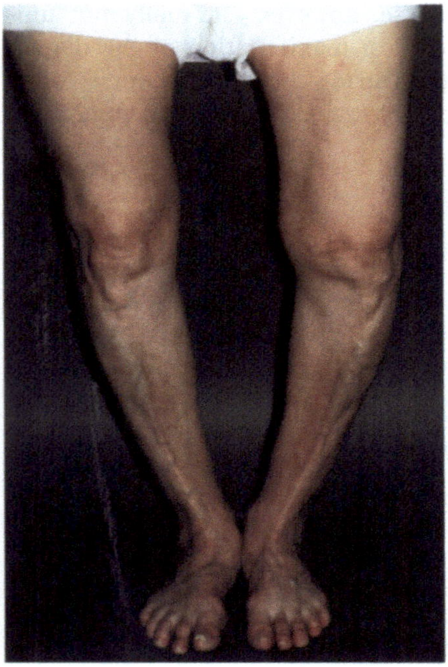

Fig. 3. Osteoarthrotic joint deformity in severe varus gonarthrosis

amplified symptoms when secondary inflammatory processes lead to an activation of the disease.

To a certain degree, the organism is able to compensate for the results of attrition. When such changes have progressed to a certain point, however, the body's ability to compensate decreases and, gradually or acutely triggered by overloading or trauma, decompensation of the precariously maintained articular balance occurs and symptoms and functional disturbances develop. Such a situation may be temporary or may initiate a permanent, sometimes rapidly progressive, complex pattern of complaints.

These observations show that both the osteoarthrotic process and its outcome are multidimensional. Depending on the severity of the disease and also whether only a single joint or a number of joints are involved, various dimensions need to be taken into account.

The observation that pain, functional loss, and morphological changes to a joint - as seen on radiograph - often do not appear to correlate should not be a surprise when we remember that the morphological changes represent merely a historical development of a process that has been ongoing over a period of many years. For practical day-to-day purposes, this means that we need to see pain and functional loss separately from anatomical and radiological changes.

The underlying causes of pain in osteoarthrosis have still not been adequately explained. From the pathophysiological point of view, increased pressure on subchondral bone, periarticular problems, synovitis and changes to the joint capsule would appear to be of relevance. However, studies in large populations have shown that pain is also determined by the general state of the patient's health, psychosocial factors and on the extent of radiological changes (Dieppe 1995).

Loss of function may be based on a multiplicity of joint-related factors. Here, a major role is played by the limitation of joint movement, the development of contractures, and loss of joint stability. As in the case of pain, however, data obtained in large studies of patients with diseases of the knee joints reveal a number of interesting details. Apparently, both the loss of power of the quadriceps muscle, and the patient's subjective awareness of pain are critical determinants of the extent of functional impairment (Dieppe 1995).

Pathogenesis of Osteoarthrosis – Clinical Aspects

Increasingly, osteoarthrosis is now being viewed not so much as a distinct entity but as a group of "overlapping" illnesses. According to this view we should thus regard the "osteoarthrotic diseases" as a group of illnesses in which the normal state of equilibrium between anabolic and catabolic processes within the articular cartilage and subchondral bone has, for a variety of reasons, broken down. This, in turn, leads to destruction of the cartilage and characteristic changes to the subchondral bone (Dieppe 1995). Such a definition recognizes the fact that osteoarthrosis is a process rather than a disease entity. The degree to which this process then manifests clinically in the form of movement-related pain and loss of normal joint function may vary enormously.

The question as to how the process is initiated continues to generate a large number of hypotheses. These range from the notion that osteoarthrosis is a mechanically induced organic failure (Felson 1995) to the belief that it is due largely to constitutional factors. Other authors consider osteoarthrosis to be a secondary consequence of a primary, generalized disease of osseous structures, rather than a cartilage disease (Dequecker et al. 1995, 1997; Radin and Rose 1986).

The concept of osteoarthrosis as a group of various illnesses derives, in the first instance, from an analysis of risk factors, and these will now be considered in more detail below.

The risk factors for hip and knee joint osteoarthrosis differ quite considerably (Dieppe 1995). Table 2 shows why these two conditions should be considered as two distinct entities within the group of osteoarthrotic diseases.

Furthermore, the distribution of risk factors for osteoarthrosis of the patello-femoral compartment in the knee joint clearly differ from that in the medial tibio-femoral compartment. The pattern of disease in the patello-femoral compartment is more closely associated with a familial predisposition and nodules in the hand, while the medial tibio-femoral variant is very often associated with obesity and prior surgery. This has led to a differentiation of the two major forms of knee joint arthrosis, MOAK and POAK (medial and patello-femoral osteoarthrosis of the knee, respectively) (Dieppe 1995).

Analysis of the risk factors also led to the pathogenetic model of arthrosis developed by Dieppe (1995). This model clearly demonstrates the interactions between a systemic predisposition to this disease, and the effects of local biomechanical factors (Fig. 4). The constitutional factors

Table 2. Comparison of the risk factors for hip and knee joint osteoarthrosis (OA) (Dieppe 1995)

Risk factors	Hip joint OA	Knee joint OA
Age	20–70 years	Usually 40–60 years
Sex	Male = Female	Female ≫ Male
Race	Rare in Asiatics	Common in black-Americans
Dysplasia	++	±
Injuries	±	++
Farm work	++	–
Squatting	–	++

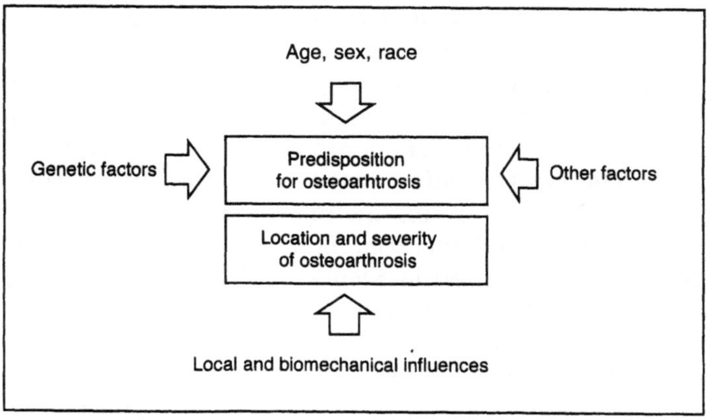

Fig. 4. Etiopathogenesis of osteoarthrosis (Dieppe 1995)

play a major role in initiating osteoarthrosis, while its location and severity is determined for the most part by local biomechanical factors.

While osteoarthrosis is a common disease, it typically affects only a few joints. A number of theories have been advanced to explain this fact. One suggestion is that the most likely sites are those joints which must be considered to have been less than optimally "planned" by the evolutionary process. On the basis of an analysis of osteoarthrosis of the wrist and hip joints, it has been shown that our joints are not adequately adapted either to an upright gait, or to the grasping function of the hand. As result, it is claimed, arthrotic changes are very frequently concentrated in the hip and the base of the thumb. Other theories, in contrast, suggest that the parts of our joints that are "insufficiently used" are most likely to develop arthrosis. Investigations performed on old skeletons provide interesting findings suggesting that MOAK was far less common among our ancestors than POAK or osteoarthrosis of the hip. These observations indicate that the present-day high incidence of osteoarthrosis – at least at some sites – may be associated with certain aspects of modern life, for example, increased obesity, or the manner in which we now make use of our joints (Dieppe 1995).

Nodal Osteoarthrosis

In the current discussions about the pathological entity, osteoarthrosis, the term nodal osteoarthrosis, to which Jones et al. (1995) attach particular importance, is receiving increasing attention. Nodal generalized osteoarthrosis (NGOA) is considered to be a special subgroup of the widely differing forms of osteoarthrosis. It is characterized by a polyarticular involvement of the hand, an early inflammatory component, Heberden and Bouchard nodes and a familial predisposition. Furthermore, nodal osteoarthrosis is associated with a concentric pattern of hip joint involvement and certain immunohistochemical findings in the arthrotic synovium and cartilage. In many women there is a dominant, in men a recessive, hereditary factor. The symptomatic form is more common in women in whom it occurs in particular around the menopause.

With regard to possible genetic markers, nodal generalized osteoarthrosis is associated with an increased incidence of HLA-A1, B8, the MZ alpha-1-antitrypsin phenotypes, and an increased incidence of homozygotic alpha-antichymotrypsin genes. Furthermore, in comparison with other forms of osteoarthrosis, nodal arthrosis is associated with an increase in IgG rheumatoid factors, lower mean levels of IgA, and an elevated prevalence of antithyroglobulin antibodies. These findings have led to the view that immunological processes are involved in the pathogenesis of this form of arthrosis. Jones et al. (1995) reported that generalized osteoarthrosis is characterized radiologically by at least grade 2 osteophyte formation in the interphalangeal joint of the thumb, and the distal interphalangeal joints of the fingers, with involvement of only a few joints.

Aging and Osteoarthrosis

Age is a strong predictor of osteoarthrosis (Mankin et al. 1986). While osteoarthrosis rarely occurs in the young, the rate increases with age. The mechanisms behind this presumably are based on the cumulative effects of loading, trauma, metabolic endocrine and other factors acting on a joint throughout the course of a lifespan. There seems to be a considerable individual variability in the rate and nature of age-related changes to the cartilage. Some of these changes must be considered benign, with no tendency to progress, while others can relatively quickly lead to the development of osteoarthrosis (Mankin et al. 1986).

Trauma and Osteoarthrosis

It is well known that injury to the joint including damage to the ligamentous structures, surface of the cartilage, the menisci and the subchondral bone can lead to osteoarthrosis. The rate and severity of the development of osteoarthrosis depends on the extent of the primary trauma and its treatment (e.g. joint incongruity caused by a fracture, instability), the localization (main loading zone, marginal zone), the importance of the traumatized structures and the ability of the organism to compensate the trauma, as also on future loading of the injured joint (occupation, sports, weight-bearing joint, non-weight-bearing joint) (Carman et al. 1994; Neyret et al. 1994; Sahlstrom and Montgomery 1997). Roos et al. (1998) for example, reported a relative risk for the development of a tibio-femoral osteoarthrosis following surgical removal of the meniscus to be 14% after 21 years.

Sports and Osteoarthrosis

Current investigations of the question as to whether sporting activities may cause osteoarthrosis raises a number of interesting questions. Lane (1995) and Buckwalter (1997) observed that healthy joints normally tolerate homogeneous sport-related loading with no negative consequences or accelerated rates of development of osteoarthrosis. Joints with prior trauma to ligaments, tendons or menisci, or with abnormal articular anatomy, as also those of persons practicing competition-level sports with a particularly high impact on the joints, appear to develop osteoarthrosis more frequently (Marti et al. 1989; Neyret et al. 1993). Sports activities involving repeated non-physiological loading peaks or torsional loads over the long-term increase the predisposition for the development of osteoarthrosis. On the other hand, it has been noted that running does not increase the risk of osteoarthrosis of the knee joint in normal recreational sports activities. In competitive sports, the risk of developing an osteoarthrosis over the long-term is, in contrast, clearly elevated (Lane 1995). This also applies to soccer and baseball players, with more or less marked differences between recreational and competitive sport (Table 3). If, however, degenerative articular changes are already present, the risk of osteoarthrosis increases even for recreational sports activities that go beyond normal day-to-day activities.

Weight and Osteoarthrosis

A review by Felson (1995) that considers the relationship between weight and osteoarthrosis notes that being overweight is a very important risk factor for osteoarthrosis of the knee and hip joint and, surprisingly, of the hand. Apparently, both local and systemic factors are involved. Women with a body mass index (BMI) of 30–35 kg/m^2, have an osteoarthrosis risk that is 4 times as high as that of women with a BMI of less than 25 kg/m^2; in the case of men with similar BMI figures the risk for gonarthrosis is 4.8 times as high (Anderson and Felson 1988).

Obesity is also associated with an increased risk of osteoarthrosis of the hip joint (Cooper et al. 1998). The association between weight and os-

Table 3. Osteoarthrosis (OA) and exercise: possible associations (Lane 1995)

	Sport	Site	Risk of OA
Normal joints	Running		
	Recreational	Knee, hip	No increase
	Competitive		Possibly increased
	Soccer		
	Recreational	Knee, ankle	No increase
	Competitive		Possibly increased
	Baseball		
	Recreational	Elbow, shoulder	No increase
	Competitive		Possibly increased
Abnormal joints	Running	Knee	Probably increased
	Soccer	Knee	Probably increased
	Football	Knee	Probably increased

teoarthrosis of the hip is, however, not as clear-cut as in the case of the knee. A possible explanation for this is that while walking the knee joint is subjected to loads of up to 6 times body weight compared with only three times the body weight for the hip. This means that the effect of weight on the knee joint is twice that on the hip.

It has been shown that overweight women who lose weight can reduce their risk of developing symptomatic osteoarthrosis – in particular of the knee joint – later in life. With an average weight loss of 11 lbs, the risk of developing clinically relevant osteoarthrosis of the knee decreased by more than 50% (Felson et al. 1992). Conversely, an increase in weight over the long-term was associated with an increase in the rate of knee joint osteoarthrosis. When osteoarthrosis is already present, the overweight are also at increased risk of disease progression, and have a more unfavorable prognosis with regard to its severity (Heppt et al. 1990).

The specific question as to why obesity is associated not only with osteoarthrosis of the knee and hip – which would have been expected – but also with an increase in osteoarthrosis of the hands (Carman et al. 1994), is currently under discussion. In overweight persons, a systemic factor (possibly a circulating cartilage growth factor or a bone factor) that accelerates cartilage breakdown resulting in osteoarthrosis is presumed to be present (Felson et al. 1992). In particular, in postmenopausal women, who are at highest risk of developing osteoarthrosis, adipose tissue may be metabolically active. Added to this, persons with obesity may have a higher bone mineral density, which, of itself may be a risk for osteoarthrosis. Since the knee joint is particularly affected in overweight persons, it may be noted that the factors of being overweight and excessive loading – possibly in combination with a systemic factor – are major determinants in the development of osteoarthrosis.

Occupational Aspects and Osteoarthrosis

Cooper (1995) reported an association between occupational joint stresses and the risk of osteoarthrosis and estimated the relative percentage of osteoarthrosis caused by occupational stresses to be about 5%.

Occupational physical stress is one of the major factors influencing in particular the development of osteoarthrosis of the knee and hip joints (Cooper 1995). A number of studies have provided data showing that occupational activities associated with frequent or prolonged squatting and heavy physical work are associated with a higher rate of knee joint osteoarthrosis (Kellgren and Lawrence 1952; Lindberg and Montgomery 1987; Partridge and Duthie 1968; Wickstrom et al. 1983). The Framingham Study (Felson et al. 1991) also showed, in a follow-up study involving 1400 persons, that the risk of osteoarthrosis was highest in persons with such occupational stresses. In all these studies, no increase was found in osteoarthrosis risk associated with job-related prolonged walking, standing, sitting or driving.

In a case-control study, Coggon et al. (1998) found a significant increase in the rate of hip joint osteoarthrosis in men whose jobs involved the lifting of heavy weights. In several studies, a particular prevalence of hip joint osteoarthrosis has been reported for farmers who, in comparison with a male population of the same age group have a tenfold higher risk of developing osteoarthrosis. Why this should be so is not at all clear, and is presently being investigated in ongoing studies. It does, however, appear that the particular physical stresses associated with such work have a major role to play (Cooper 1995; Croft et al. 1992; Vingard et al. 1990).

Nutrition and Osteoarthrosis

Nutritional influences on the development of osteoarthrosis still remain unclear (McAlindon and Felson 1997). There is, however, evidence that such factors also play an etiological role in osteoarthrosis. Thus, a diet rich in vitamin C appears to have a protective effect against the destruction of cartilage in the guinea pig osteoarthrosis model (Meacock et al. 1990). In the Framingham Knee OA Cohort Study, however, no significant relationship was found between the intake of antioxidant micronutrients (vitamin C, vitamin E and beta carotene) and the incidence of radiographic knee joint osteoarthrosis (McAlindon et al. 1996b). One of the causes of the low incidence of hip joint arthrosis in the Chinese is considered to be their low-calorie diet. Experimentally induced vitamin B6 deficiency led to lesions of the cartilage similar to those seen in osteoarthrosis. In epidemiological studies, McAlindon et al. (1996a) found an association between low serum levels of vitamin D and an increased incidence of knee joint osteoarthrosis. In the case of the Kashin-Beck disease (endemic arthrosis deformans), nutritional factors are assumed to play a role (Mathieu et al. 1997).

There exist indications that nutritional factors can influence the course of osteoarthrosis through a variety of mechanisms. Overall, however, it must be admitted that we still have no certain knowledge of the influence of dietary factors on the development of osteoarthrosis.

Conclusions

In summary, currently available epidemiological data show that the major non-constitutional risk factors for knee joint osteoarthrosis are obesity, previous injury to the knee joint, meniscectomy, occupation-related excessive loading of the knee joint, and the presence of Heberden's nodes. The risk profile for hip joint osteoarthrosis deviates somewhat from that of knee joint osteoarthrosis. Although there is a relationship between osteoarthrosis and overweight, prior injury to the hip and the presence of Heberden's nodes, it is less obvious in the case of the knee. Additional aspects are local biomechanical influences and endogenous factors the interactions of which may initiate the process of osteoarthrosis.

For practical purposes, all this means that osteoarthrosis should by no means be considered to be a single-dimensional, monocausal entity, and certainly not an unavoidable stroke of fate.

The clinical course of this condition is extremely variable in terms of its manifestation and individual symptoms. As a result, an individual consideration of the symptoms and functional deficits of a given patient is much more important than any evaluation based on pathomorphological changes.

In addition to a specific therapy, modifications to lifestyle and ambient conditions offer numerous possibilities for influencing the course of the disease and its symptoms. In view of this, it is of particular importance for the clinician to be familiar with all the factors involved, and to give due consideration to them when planning his treatment strategy. The early elimination of risk factors, early diagnosis and surveillance of the disease and appropriate treatment of pain and functional deficits offer effective means of prevention and treatment in the various stages of the osteoarthrotic disease process.

References

Andersen J, Felson DT (1988) Factors associated with osteoarthritis of the knee in the first national health and nutrition examination survey (HANES I). Am J Epidemiol 128:179–189

Boszotta H, Helperstorfer W, Kolndorder G (1994) Long-term results of arthroscopic meniscectomy. Aktuelle Traumatol 24:30–34

Buckwalter JA, Martin JA (1995) Degenerative joint disease. In: Clinical symposia. Ciba-Geigy, Summit, New Jersey, pp 2–32
Buckwalter JA, Lane NE (1997) Athletics and osteoarthritis. Am J Sports Med 25:873–881
Buckwalter JA, Mankin HJ (1997) Articular cartilage. Part II. Degeneration and osteoarthrosis, repair, regeneration and transplantation. J Bone Joint Surg 79-A4:612–632
Carman WJ, Sowers MF, Hawthorne VM, Weissfeld LA (1994) Obesity as a risk factor of osteoarthritis of the hand and wrist: a prospective study. Am J Epidemiol 139:119–129
Coggon D, Kellingray S, Inkip H, Croft P, Campbell L, Cooper C (1998) Osteoarthritis of the hip and occupational lifting. Am J Epidemiol 147:523–528
Cooper C (1995) Occupational activity and the risk of osteoarthritis. J Rheumatol 22 [Suppl 43]:10–12
Cooper C, Inskip H, Croft P, Campbell L, Smith G, McLaren M, Coggon D (1998) Individual risk factors for hip osteoarthritis: obesity, hip injury and physical activity. Am J Epidemiol 147:516–522
Croft P, Coggon D, Cruddas M, Cooper C (1992) Osteoarthritis of the hip: an occupational disease in farmers. BMJ 304:1269–1272
Dieppe P (1995) Auf der Suche nach einer wirksamen Therapie der Arthrose. Primäre, sekundäre und tertiäre Prävention. Rheumatologie in Europa 24:118–121
Dieppe P (1995) Arthrose: Risikofaktoren, Therapie und Ausgang. Rheumatologie in Europa 24:66–68
Dequecker J, Mokassa L, Aerssens J (1995) Bone density and osteoarthritis. J Rheumatol 22 [Suppl 43]:98–100
Dequecker J, Mokassa L, Aerssens J, Boonen S (1997) Bone density and local growth factors in generalized osteoarthritis. Microsc Res Tech 37:358–371
Felson DT, Hannan MT, Nairmark A, Berkeley J, Gordon G, Wilson PW, Anderson J (1991) Occupational physical demands, knee bending and knee osteoarthritis: results from the Framingham study. J Rheumatol 18:1587–1592
Felson DT, Ahange Y, Anthony JM, Nairmark A, Anderson JJ (1992) Weight loss reduces the risk for symptomatic knee osteoarthritis in women. Ann Intern Med 116:535–539
Felson DT (1995) Weight and osteoarthritis. J Rheumatol 22 [Suppl 43]:7–9
Heppt P, Goldmann A, Beyer W, Wirtz P (1990) Indications, risks and long-term results of high tibial barrel-vault ostetomy. Orthop Praxis 26:106–109
Jones AC, Hopkinson ND, Pattrick M, Doherty M (1995) Die nodale Arthrose: Welches Ausmaß an radiographisch gesicherter Arthrose ist erforderlich um den Komplex zu definieren? Rheumatologie in Europa 24:115–117
Kellgren JH, Lawrence JS (1952) Rheumatism in miners. Part II. X-ray study. Br J Indust Med 9:197–207
Lane NE (1995) Exercise: a cause of osteoarthritis. J Rheumatol 22 [Suppl 43]:3–6
Lindberg H, Montgomery F (1987) Heavy labour and the occurrence of gonarthrosis. Clin Orthop 214:235–236
Mankin HJ, Brandt KD, Shulman LE (1986) Workshop on ethiopathogenesis of osteoarthritis. Proceedings and recommendations. J Rheumatol 13:1130–1148
Marti B, Knobloch M, Tschopp A, Jucker A, Howald A (1989) Is excessive running predictive of degenerative hip disease? Controlled study of former elite athletes. BMJ 299:91–93
Mathieu F, Begaux F, Lan ZY, Suetens C, Hinsenkamp M (1997) Clinical manifestations of Kashin-Beck disease in Nyemo Valley, Tibet. Int Orthop 21:151–156
McAlindon TE, Felson DT, Zhang Y, Hannan MT, Alibadi P, Weissman B, Rush D, Wilson PW, Jaques P (1996a) Relation of dietary intake and serum levels of vitamin D to progression of osteoarthritis of the knee among participants in the Framingham study. Ann Intern Med 125:353–359

McAlindon TE, Jacques T, Zhang Y, Hannan MT, Alibadi P, Weissman B (1996b) Do antioxidant micronutrients protect against the development and the progression of knee osteoarthritis. Arthritis Rheum 39:648–656

McAlindon TE, Felson DT (1997) Nutrition: risk factors for osteoarthritis. Ann Rheum Dis 56:3397–3400

Meacock SCR, Bodmer JL, Billingham MEJ (1990) Experimental OA in guinea pigs. J Exp Pathol 71:279–293

Neyret P, Donell ST, DeJour P, DeJour H (1993) Partial meniscectomy and anterior cruciate ligament rupture in soccer players. A study with a minimum 20-year follow-up. Am J Sports Med 21:455–460

Neyret P, Donell ST, DeJour H (1994) Osteoarthritis of the knee following meniscectomy. Br J Rheumatol 33:267–268

Partridge REH, Duthie JJR (1968) Rheumatism in dockers and civil servants: a comparison of heavy manual and sedentary workers. Ann Rheum Dis 27:559–568

Radin EL, Rose RM (1986) Role of subchondral bone in the initiation and progression of cartilage damage. Clin Orthop 213:34–40

Roos H, Lauren M, Adalberth T, Roos EM, Jonsson K, Lohmander LS (1998) Knee osteoarthritis after meniscectomy: prevalence of radiographic changes after twenty-one years, compared with matched controls. Arthritis Rheum 41:687–693

Sahlstrom A, Montgomery F (1997) Risk analysis of occupational factors influencing the development of arthrosis of the knee. Eur J Epidemiol 13:675–679

Vingard E, Alfredsson L, Goldie I, Hogstedt C (1990) Occupation and osteoarthritis of the hip and knee: a register-based cohort study. Int J Epidemiol 20:1025–1031

Wickstrom G, Haninen K, Mattsson T et al. (1983) Knee degeneration in concrete reinforcement workers. Br J Indust Med 40:216–219

Morphogenesis of Osteoarthrosis

W. Mohr

Introduction

The different morphological aspects of osteoarthrosis, especially the disease modifying secondary and tertiary events, indicating that joint failure is more than cartilage loss, may be demonstrated by a short case report.

The 64-year-old female patient presented here suffered from "monarthritis" of the hip joint. By nuclear magnetic resonance "synovial proliferation" and bone marrow edema of the femoral head were diagnosed. A tentative diagnosis of "foudroyant" osteoarthrosis was made; nevertheless, this diagnosis seemed not to be supported by the observed synovial proliferation. A synovial biopsy showed a marked debris synovitis with fragments of cartilage and bone enclosed in synovial villi. This histological finding led to the assumption that the clinical symptoms were due to osteoarthrosis with secondary ischemic bone necrosis.

The operative specimen supported this idea. Macroscopically the femoral head showed an advanced cartilage loss (Fig. 1 a). Histologically, remnants of fibrillated cartilage covered the periphery of the specimen (Fig. 1 b). Sections from the insertion region of the ligamentum capitis femoris (Fig. 1 a) exhibited necrotic bone with adjacent granulation tissue and chondroid tissue (Fig. 1c, d). As seen in the biopsy, the villous synovial tissue contained fragments of bone and cartilage (Fig. 1 e and f) supporting the previous diagnosis of debris synovitis. From the pathological point of view the different aspects of the disease were understandable.

This case report leads to the conclusion that it may be wise to differentiate primary, secondary and even tertiary events that can occur during the development of osteoarthrotic joint failure (Fig. 2).

Primary Event: Cartilage Destruction

Several hypotheses are discussed to explain the disease initiating cartilage loss. According to Dean (1991) there is no doubt that metalloproteinases of the chondrocytes "digest" the extracellular matrix. On the

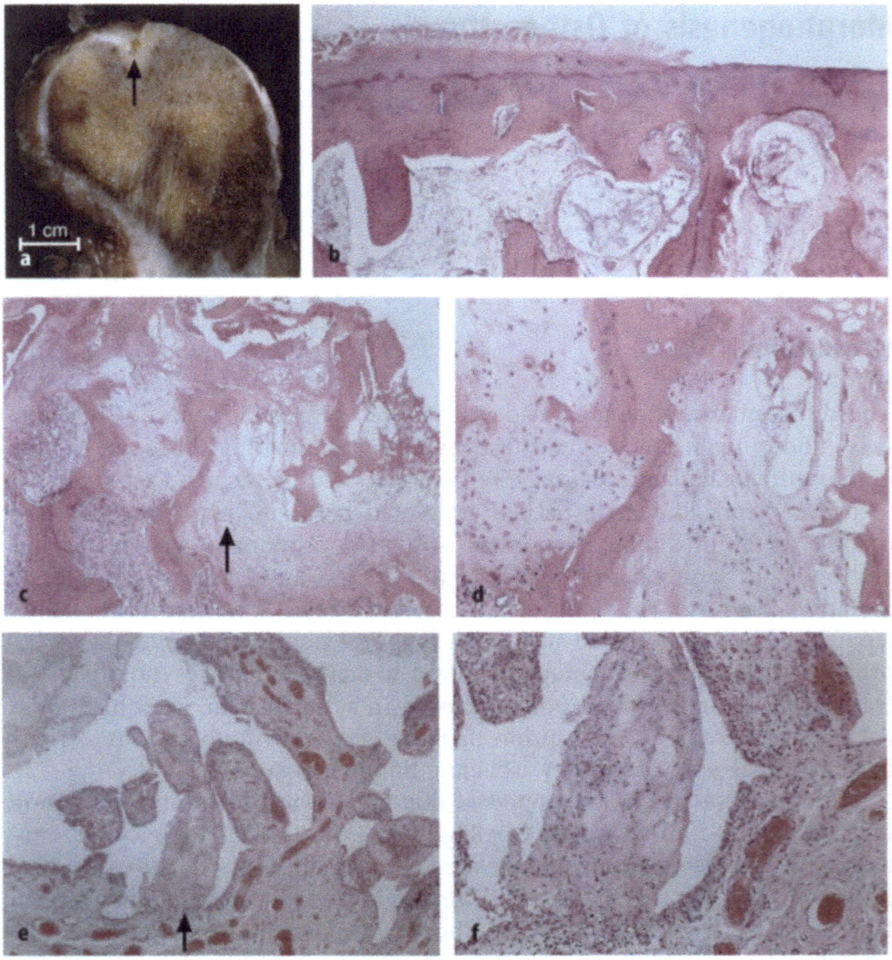

Fig. 1 a–f. *Advanced osteoarthrosis of the femoral head.* **a** Femoral head with peripheral remnants of cartilage. Arrow indicates insertion of the ligamentum capitis femoris. **b** Remnants of fibrillated cartilage bordering on denuded bone hematoxylin eosin HE, 30:1. **c** From the insertion of the ligamentum capitis femoris (*arrow in* **a**): osteonecrosis followed by granulation tissue HE, 30:1. **d** Higher magnification of **c** (*arrow*): remnants of necrotic bone surrounded by new-formed bone and chondroid tissue HE, 60:1. **e** Villous hyperplasia of the synovial membrane HE, 30:1. **f** Higher magnification of **e** (*arrow*): synovial villus with enclosed cartilage fragments HE, 60:1

other hand alterations of collagen composition, e.g. an increased synthesis of collagen type X seems possible (von der Mark et al. 1992).

The morphology renders it plausible that the initial event is the decay of chondrocytes in pressure zones, whether due to necrosis or apoptosis.

The "chondrocyte-death" hypothesis, which indicates that cell decay is induced by mechanical forces, is deduced from histological observations

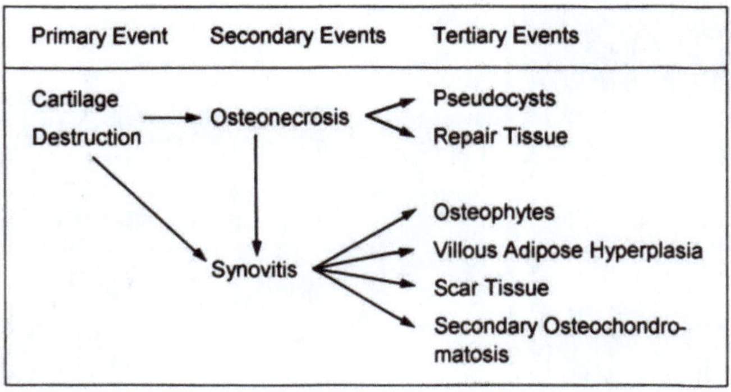

Fig. 2. Events leading to osteoarthrotic joint remodeling

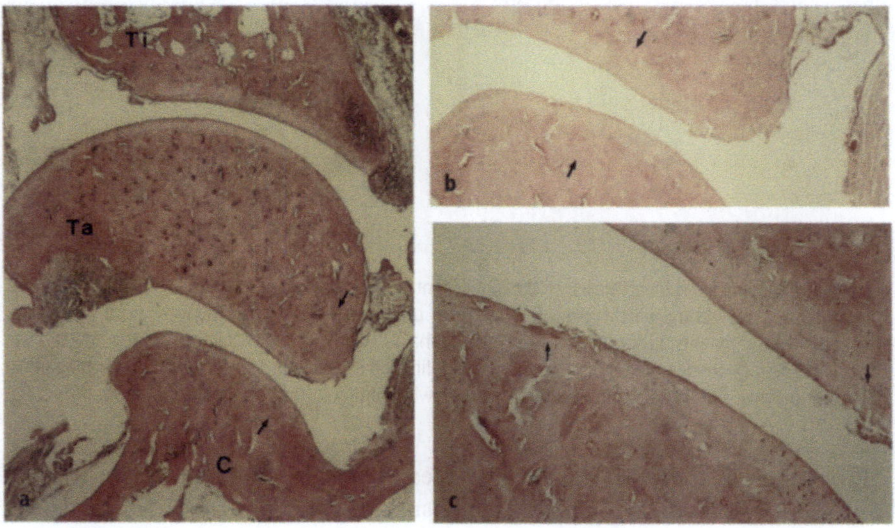

Fig. 3 a–c. Morphology of the ankle joint of an old rat demonstrating tibia (*Ti*), talus (*Ta*) and calcaneus (*C*) [from Mohr et al. (1997)]. **a** Low-power view of articulation demonstrating the two different joints and the surrounding normal uninflamed synovial tissue HE, 10:1. **b** Higher magnification of area marked by arrows in **a** focal destruction of the cartilage HE, 35:1. **c** Higher magnification of area marked by arrows in **b** focal destruction of the cartilage with chondrocytic necroses and fibrillation of matrix (*arrows*) HE, 85:1

of the ankle joints of old rats (Mohr and Lehmann 1992) – similar results were reported by Bendele and Hulman (1988) in guinea pigs with knee osteoarthrosis. Minor morphological changes in the ankle joints of these rats consist in sharply demarked cartilage areas with loss of chondrocyte nuclei and reduced stainability with safranin-O, indicating loss of proteoglycans. More advanced changes are fibrillation of the cartilage in pressure zones

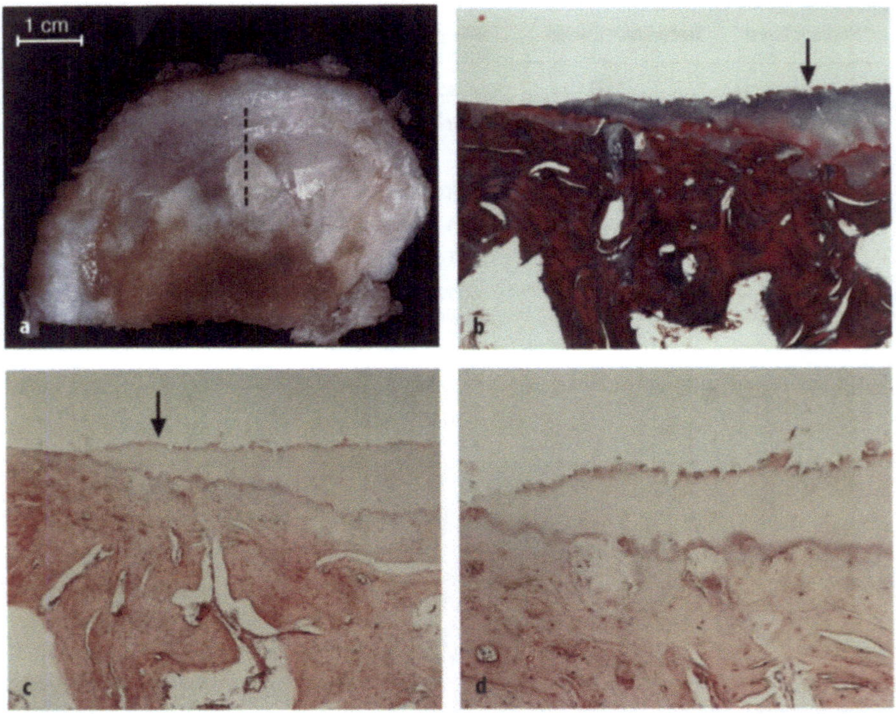

Fig. 4 a–d. Advanced osteoarthrosis of the knee joint. **a** Macroscopy of tibial plateau with remnants of cartilage in the central part. Broken line indicates origin of the histological specimen. **b** Hyperostotic bone with remnants of cartilage (*arrow*) Heidenhain's Azan, 30:1. **c** Structure of the "destructive front": bordering on denuded bone wedge-shaped fibrillated cartilage HE, 30:1. **d** Higher magnification of **c** (*arrow*): fibrillated wedge-shaped cartilage with complete loss of chondrocytes HE, 60:1

(Fig. 3 a–c), in the most advanced stages there is a complete loss of hyaline and even calcified cartilage with exposure of subchondral bone.

Similar morphological sequences can be observed in the human joints. Figure 4 a demonstrates the advanced loss of cartilage from the tibial bone of the knee joint. Histology of the "destructive front" exhibits denuded bone with remnants of cartilage in the neighborhood (Fig. 4 b), the surface of this cartilage is fibrillated, the chondrocytes have disappeared (Fig. 4 c, d).

Secondary Events

In the course of the disease secondary events develop in the subchondral bone and in the synovial membrane (Fig. 2).

Osteonecrosis

Secondary osteonecrosis may be observed in operative specimens of the knee and hip joints – nevertheless, ischemic or "aseptic" bone necrosis occurs also in other joints (Mohr 1996). In early stages of this complication the surface of the femoral head shows circumscript yellow areas in the zone of complete cartilage loss (Fig. 5a). The sectioned specimen exhibits necrosis of the subchondral bone (Fig. 5b), sometimes in a wedge-shaped fashion. Histological sections from this area show fragmented necrotic bone with loss of the osteocyte nuclei (Fig. 5c and d). A resorptive reaction has started in the neighboring bone marrow: granulation tissue occupies the intertrabecular space (Fig. 5e) and encloses fragments of bone and cartilage (Fig. 5f). Necroses of this kind have been observed in about 80% of osteoarthrotic femoral heads (Gabriel 1996).

Synovitis

It must be argued that osteoarthrosis accompanying inflammatory synovial reactions is due to erosion of cartilage and bone, especially in cases with secondary osteonecrosis. Molecular degradation products of proteoglycans, as was shown by Boniface et al. (1988) after injecting purified proteoglycans into rabbit knee joints, may induce a lymphoplasmocytic synovitis. On the other hand cartilage and bone shards induce a fibrinous synovitis: macroscopically the synovial surface is covered by a villous fibrinous exudate (Fig. 6a, b), histologically fragments of bone or cartilage can be detected in the fibrin (Fig. 6c–e). Mechanically induced vascular lesions with increased leakage of fibrinogen followed by intraarticular polymerisation may be the basic event.

Tertiary Events

Tertiary events that occur in bones and synovial tissues (see Fig. 2) are responsible for further joint remodeling.

Pseudocysts

In a morphological survey on operative specimens of osteoarthritic femoral heads, subchondral pseudocysts occurred in 73% of all cases (Fig. 7). Usually they are associated with secondary bone necrosis, necrotic bone remnants are present in their often fibrous wall (Gabriel 1996). From these observations it is concluded that osteonecrosis precedes the forma-

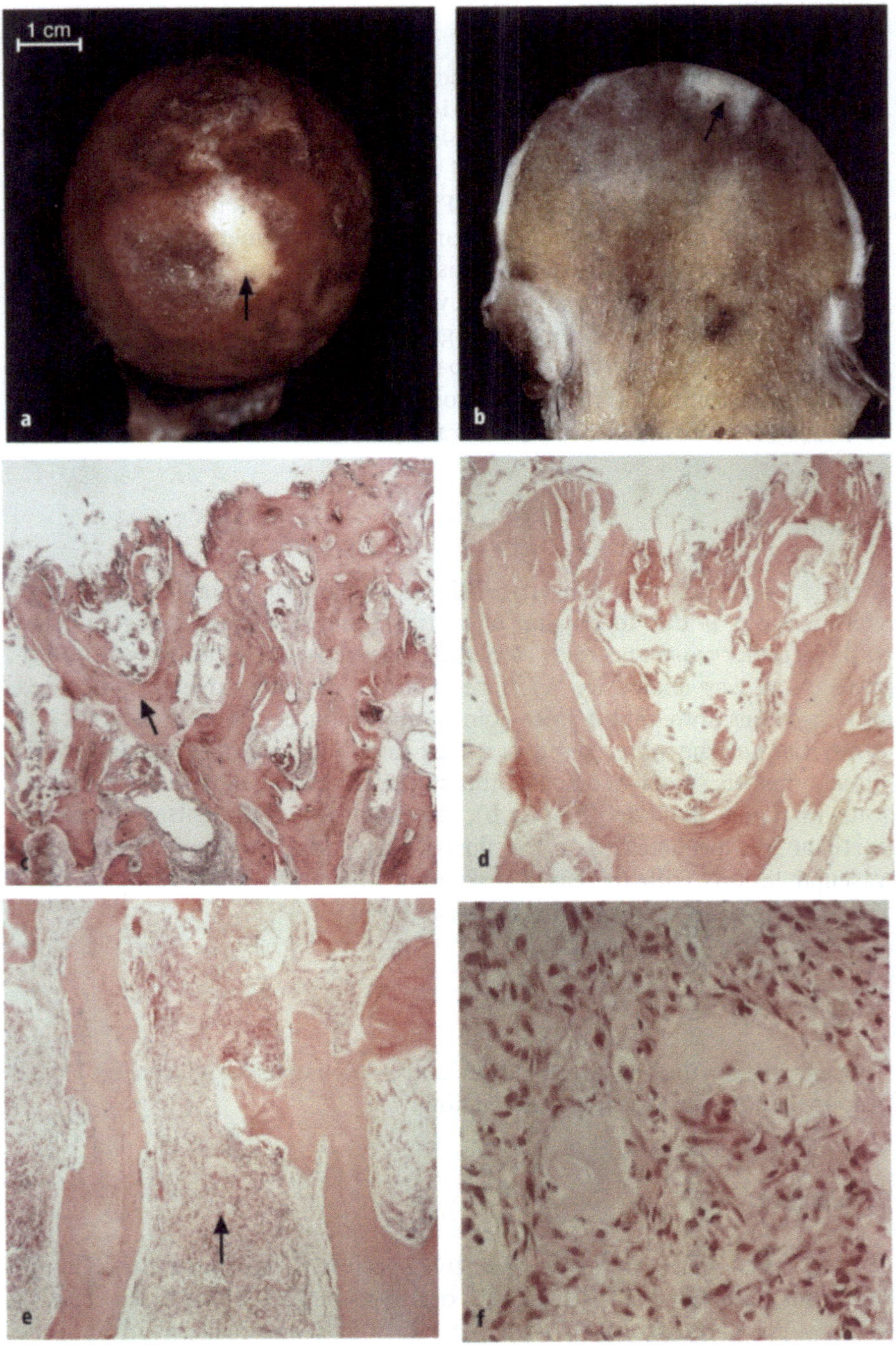
1 cm
a
b
d
e
f

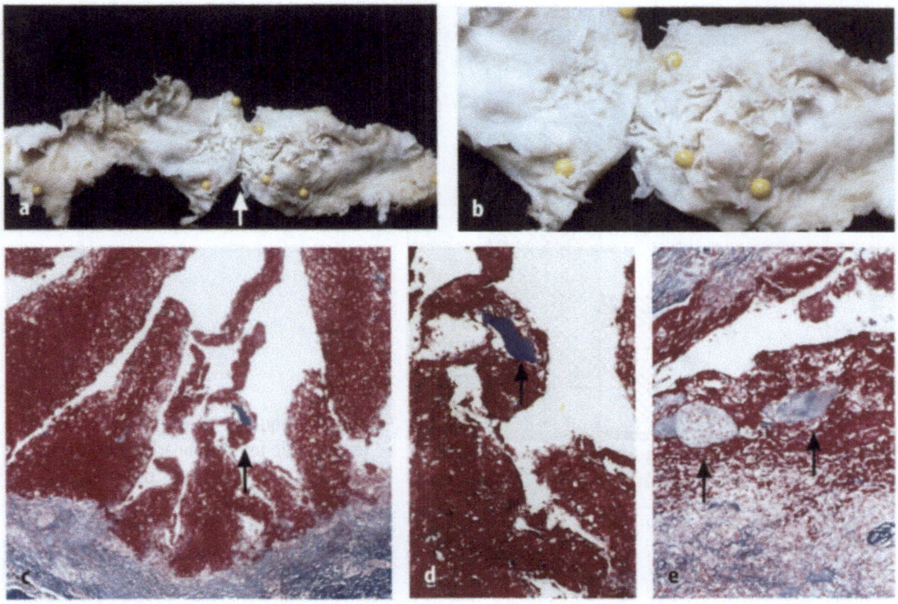

Fig. 6 a–e. Fibrinous debris-synovitis. **a** Operation specimen from the knee joint covered by villous fibrin. **b** Detail from **a** (*arrow*): synovial membrane with villous fibrin. **c** Villous fibrin covers the synovial tissue Heidenhain's Azan 30:1. **d** Higher magnification of **c** (*arrow*): cartilage fragment (*arrow*) surrounded by fibrin Heidenhain's Azan, 60:1. **e** Fibrinous exudate with cartilage fragments (*arrows*) and granulation tissue invading the fibrin Heidenhain's Azan, 60:1

tion of these geodes. Intrusion of synovial fluid from the joint cavity through minor bone defects in the necrotic zones may be the morphogenetic factor.

Localization and macroscopic morphology of these pseudocysts are documented in Fig. 8: they occur preferentially in the cartilage denuded area (Fig. 8 a, c, d), sometimes they are located at the basis of necrotic bone (Fig. 8 b), and geodes may be solitary (Fig. 8 c) or multiple (Fig. 8 a, d).

◄

Fig. 5 a–f. Secondary ischemic osteonecrosis in advanced osteoarthrosis. **a** Surface of femoral head with yellow area (*arrow*). **b** "Saw-section" from the area indicated by arrow in **a**: superficial osteonecrosis (*arrow*). **c** Histology from **b** (*arrow*) necrotic bone with disrupted surface HE, 30:1. **d** Higher magnification of **c** (*arrow*) disrupted necrotic bone HE, 60:1. **e** Resorptive reaction in the neighborhood of osteonecrosis: granulation tissue in the marrow space HE, 60:1. **f** Higher magnification of **e** (*arrow*) granulation tissue surrounds fragments of cartilage HE, 180:1

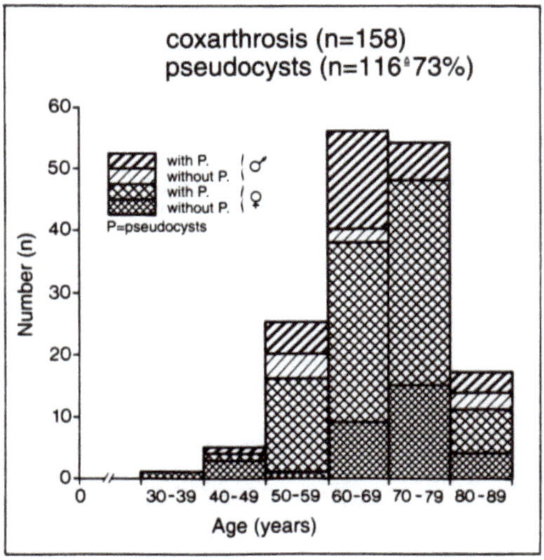

Fig. 7. Frequency of pseudocysts in osteoarthrotic femoral heads of different age classes (*with P,* with pseudocysts, *without P,* without pseudocysts)

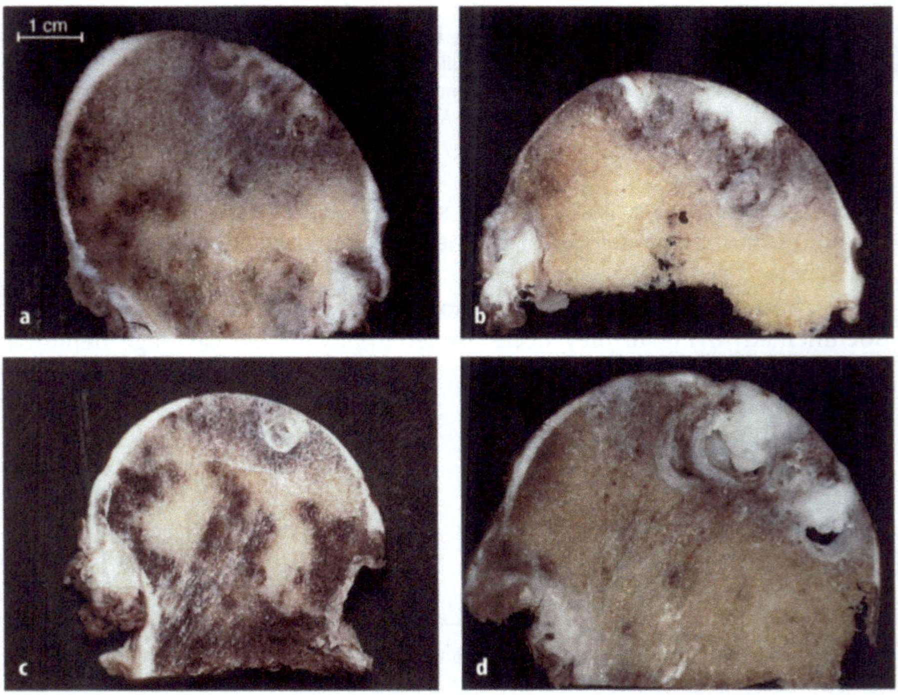

Fig. 8 a–d. Macroscopic appearance of "geodes" in the denuded bone of the weight-bearing area of the femoral head. **a** Multiple pseudocysts. **b** Pseudocysts at the basis of osteonecrosis. **c** Solitary pseudocyst. **d** Pseudocysts filled with remnants of necrotic tissue

Repair Tissue

Bone necroses with defects of the overlying osseous tissue are usually sites of the development of different kinds of repair tissues. As in Pridie's drilling (1959; Baldovin et al. 1997) granulation tissue develops from the subchondral bone marrow and grows onto the surface. Presumably under the influence of pressure this early reparative tissue is transformed into chondroid tissue that later on covers the surface of the bone in a mushroom-like fashion or occupies huge areas of the surface (Fig. 9a). The histological equivalent is chondroid tissue that borders on the subchondral bone without any tidemark (Fig. 9b). Chondroid tissue just in the neighborhood of the subchondral bone may be rich in proteoglycans as evidenced by the stainability with safranin-O (Fig. 9c).

Osteophytes

The pathogenesis of one of the most remarkable radiological signs of the disease, the osteophytes, has to be regarded in conjunction with the synovial inflammation. Figure 10 summarizes the events leading to these bony spurs.

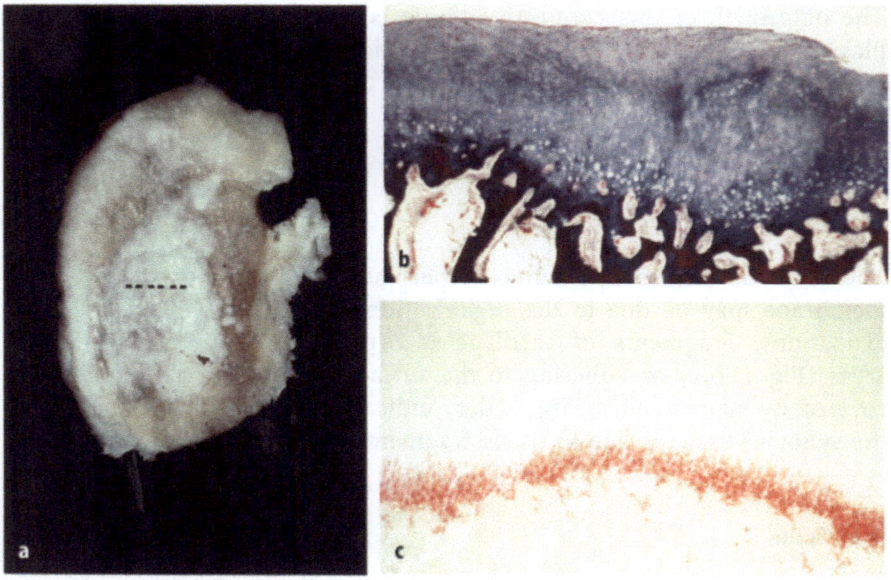

Fig. 9a–c. Chondroid repair tissue covering osteoarthrotic femoral condyle. **a** Chondroid tissue surrounded by denuded bone. Broken line indicates origin of the histological specimen. **b** Chondroid tissue covering bone Heidenhain's Azan, 30:1. **c** Demonstration of proteoglycan content of the basic chondroid tissue safranin-O, 30:1

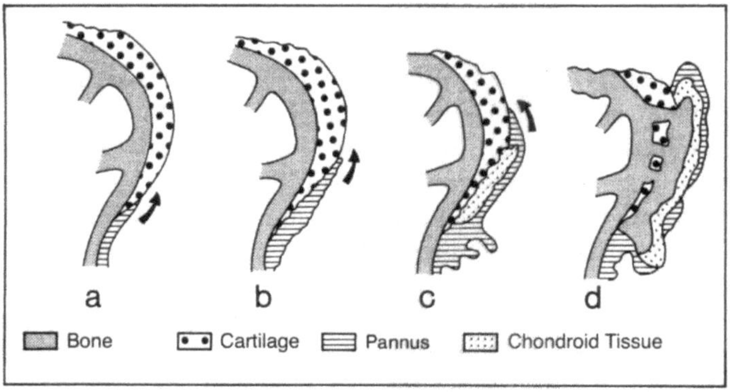

Fig. 10 a–d. Schematic representation of morphogenesis of osteophytes (according to Mohr and Regel [1985]). **a** Early proliferation of pannus tissue. **b** More advanced pannus tissue covers marginal cartilage. **c** Chondroid metaplasia in advanced pannus tissue. **d** Advanced osteophyte with superficial pannus tissue, chondroid tissue and new-formed bone covers remnants of the "buried" hyaline cartilage

As in primary inflammatory joint diseases, e.g. rheumatoid arthritis, a growing pannus tissue develops that covers the cartilage. The lack of neutrophilic granulocytes in this tissue in osteoarthrosis may explain its limited destructive capacity with regard to the underlying hyaline cartilage. The outgrowth of this connective tissue is followed by chondroid metaplasia and subsequent enchondral ossification. As a consequence the original hyaline cartilage may be surrounded or "buried" by these bone excrescenses.

Villous Adipose Hyperplasia

The focal or diffuse lipomatous hyperplasia (Fig. 11 a) of the synovial membrane may be due to the organization of previous villous fibrinous exudations. Fragments of cartilage incorporated in superficial fibrous areas (Fig. 11 b, c) or adhering to the surface of adipose villi, sometimes covered by synoviocytes (Fig. 11 d, e) indicate that this transformation of the synovial tissue is due to tissue fragments.

Scar Tissue

Scarring of the synovial tissue may occur: fibrous villi or a flattened fibrous synovial membrane has developed. Fragments of bone and cartilage in this tissue also indicate that they are responsible for this transformation.

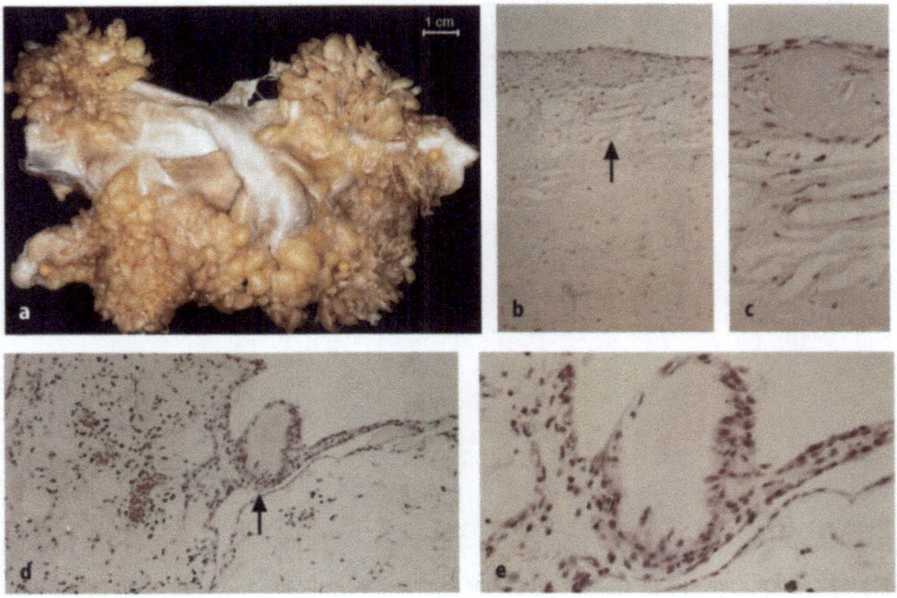

Fig. 11 a–e. Villous adipose hyperplasia of synovial membrane. **a** Operation specimen of the knee joint exhibiting synovial tissue with villous adipose areas. **b** Synovial membrane with enclosed cartilage fragment HE, 60:1. **c** Higher magnification of **b** (*arrow*): cartilage fragment enclosed in the synovial membrane HE, 180:1. **d** Villous adipose synovial tissue with adherent cartilage fragment HE, 60:1. **e** Higher magnification of **d** (*arrow*): cartilage fragment surrounded by synoviocytes HE, 180:1

Secondary Osteochondromatosis

Fragments of necrotic bone incorporated in the synovial tissue may induce a "bone morphogenetic" effect. Comparable to the ability of the bone morphogenetic proteins (Urist 1995), connective tissue cells may be transformed into osteoblasts with subsequent synthesis of bone matrix. Histologically, this situation is characterized by remnants of necrotic bone, more or less surrounded by newly formed woven bone (Fig. 12) with often peripherally situated osteoblasts. As in fracture healing bone new formation may also be due to enchondral ossification of metaplastic chondroid tissue. Osteomata or osteochondromata, sessile or pedunculated, may develop and interfere with the function of the joint.

In 1978 Ali wrote: "At present most research workers have their own picture of osteoarthrosis". This situation has not fundamentally changed in the past 20 years. The coming and going of hypotheses, theories, and even philosophies about one of the oldest diseases of vertebrates ranging from elephants to mice, may allow even a pathologist to have his own view on the development of this sometimes crippling disorder.

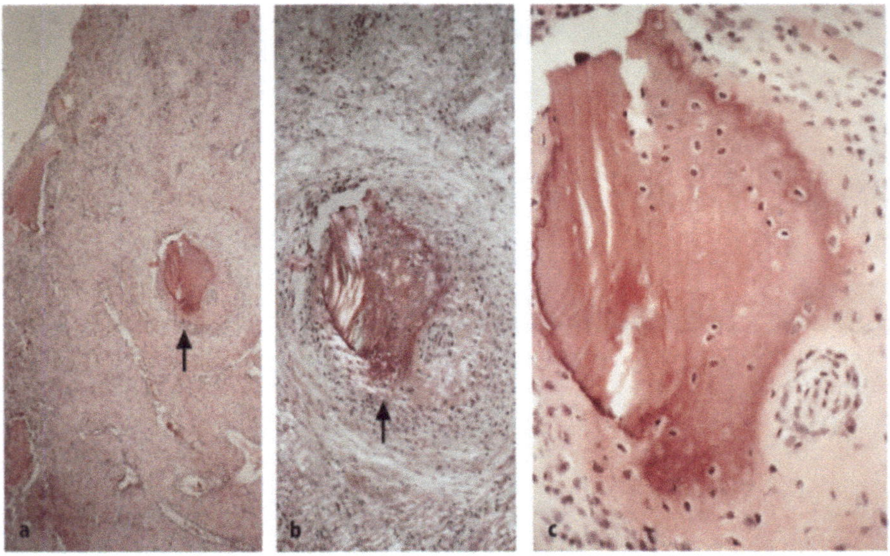

Fig. 12 a–c. Osteogenesis in synovial membrane with debris synovitis. **a** Synovial tissue with bone fragments HE, 30:1. **b** Higher magnification of **a** (*arrow*): fragment of lamellar and woven bone HE (polarized light), 60:1. **c** Higher magnification of **b** (*arrow*): necrotic lamellar bone with adjacent new-formed woven bone with osteocytes inside the matrix HE, 180:1

References

Ali SY (1978) New knowledge of osteoarthrosis. J Clin Pathol 12 [Suppl]:191–199

Baldovin M, Mariani C, Vitella A (1997) Arthroscopic abrasion arthroplasty of the knee: long-term results of 250 cases (abstract). J Bone Joint Surg 79B [Suppl II]:S176

Bendele AM, Hulman JF (1988) Spontaneous cartilage degeneration in guinea pigs. Arthritis Rheum 31:561–565

Boniface RJ, Cain PR, Evans CH (1988) Articular responses to purified cartilage proteoglycans. Arthritis Rheum 31:258–266

Dean DD (1991) Proteinase-mediated cartilage degradation in osteoarthritis. Semin Arthritis Rheum 20 [Suppl 2]:2–11

Gabriel JKP (1996) Pseudozysten – Folge primärer und sekundärer ischämischer Hüftkopfnekrosen (Dissertation). Universität Ulm, Ulm

Mohr W (1996) Pathogenese der Gelenkzerstörung bei der chronischen Polyarthritis. Radiologie 36:593–599

Mohr W, Regel E (1985) Die Entwicklung der Randexostosen bei der Koxarthrose. Aktuel Rheumatol 10:119–124

Mohr W, Lehmann H (1992) Osteoarthrosis of the ankle joint in old rats. Z Rheumatol 51:35–40

Mohr W, Lehmann H, Engelhardt G (1997) Chondroneutrality of meloxicam in rats with spontaneous osteoarthrosis of the ankle joint. Z Rheumatol 56:21–30

Pridie KH (1959) A method of resurfacing osteoarthritic knee joints. J Bone Joint Surg 41B:618–619

Urist MR (1995) The first three decades of bone morphogenetic protein research. Osteologie 4:207–223
von der Mark K, Kirsch T, Nerlich A, Kuss A, Weseloh G, Glückert K, Stöss H (1992) Type X collagen synthesis in human osteoarthritic cartilage. Indication of chondrocyte hypertrophy. Arthritis Rheum 35:806–811

Written under the sun of Limone sul Garda at 40 °C, August 1998; completed by Rosi Endres-Klein in Ulm

Movement-Induced Orientation: A Potential Mechanism of Cartilage Collagen Network Morphogenesis

K. Ito and S. Tepic

Introduction

Articular cartilage is a layer of tissue lining the articulating osseous ends in diarthroidal joints. Its primary function is to provide a durable, low friction, load-bearing surface. Cartilage on cartilage, lubricated with synovial fluid, has a coefficient of friction of 0.02–0.005 (Charnley 1959), and regularly provides problem-free performance for a lifetime. Although this may not seem so remarkable, comparison to synthetic bearings is quite revealing. The coefficient of friction for steel on steel lubricated with oil is 0.1 (Jones 1936) and that of dry Teflon on Teflon is 0.04 (Bowden and Tabor 1950). Furthermore, the life of mechanical bearings is often less than 20 years. Articular cartilage is an exceptional material with an optimal design for its function.

This superior performance of articular cartilage is due to the poroelastic nature of its abundant extracellular matrix, i.e. a mixture of solid (35–25% w/w) and fluid (65–75% w/w) (Maroudas et al. 1976; Venn and Maroudas 1977). The solid matrix is composed of a coarse fibrous network of type-II collagen within which proteoglycan (PG) aggregates form an entangled molecular network. The latter is immobilized by the collagen network, perhaps by ionic bonds (Mow et al. 1984; Nimni 1975; Orkin et al. 1976) (Fig. 1). When the joint is loaded, cartilage consolidates and exudes its interstitial matrix fluid (Fig. 2). The load is carried by fluid pressure, which is maintained through fluid flow resistance of the PG network. The low friction lubrication of the joint is also dependent on limiting fluid expression from cartilage layers. Although the collagen network itself does not appreciably resist fluid flow, it immobilizes the entangled PGs to collectively retard the movement of interstitial fluid. Thus, the collagen network architecture significantly affects cartilage mechanical properties and its function.

As expected from its unique functional properties, the collagen network architecture is highly organized. This architecture is often described by partition of the cartilage into four separate layers or zones (Weiss et al. 1968). The superficial tangential zone (STZ), nearest the articular surface, consists of collagen fibers arranged tangential to the surface with

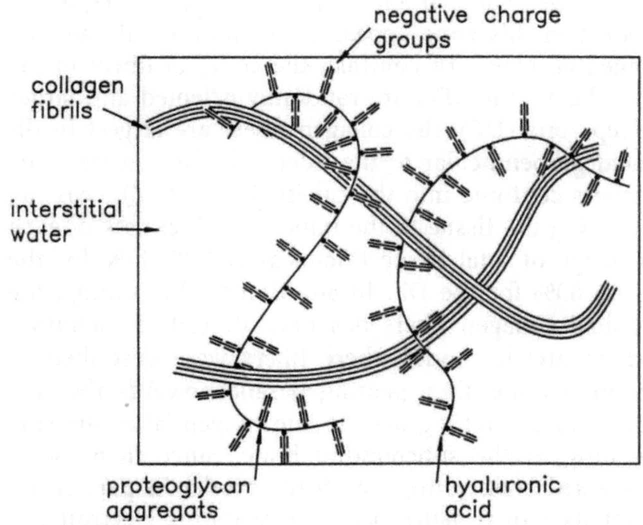

Fig. 1. Schematic representation of *unloaded* cartilage depicting a porous solid matrix of collagen and proteoglycan aggregates swollen in water

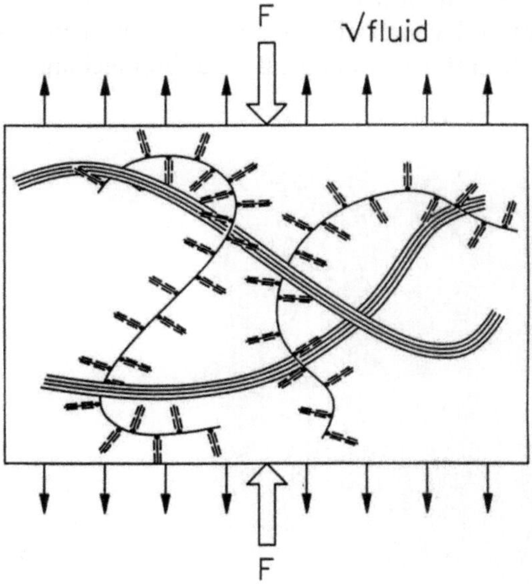

Fig. 2. Schematic representation of *loaded* cartilage depicting a porous solid matrix of collagen and proteoglycan aggregates swollen in water. *F*, applied force. √fluid, fluid velocity

the lamina splendans, a woven sheet of almost pure collagen fibers, at the actual surface. The fibers in this zone appear to be additionally aligned locally within the tangential plane. In contrast, the collagen fibers in the middle zone (MZ), just below the STZ, are randomly oriented and larger in diameter. In the deep zone (DZ), the collagen fibers are largest in diameter and are oriented perpendicular to the tidemark, the calcified cartilage border. These fibers continue into the calcified zone (CZ), crossing the tidemark and anchoring the tissue to the bone. The thickness of each zone varies: the percentage of total tissue thickness is 10%–15% for the STZ and MZ, and up to 80% for the DZ. In addition to this zoning, the organization of individual collagen fibers has been described. Benninghoff (1925) proposed an arcade model where fibers were described as arising in the subchondral bone, then passing parallel towards the surface in a radial manner before arching over to run tangential to the surface and finally returning to the subchondral bone. Since then, other models have been proposed confirming the arcade model in part (from the DZ to STZ, but not its return path), based on scanning electron microscopy investigations (Fig. 3) (Clark 1985; Kääb et al. 1996). Although it is generally accepted that this highly organized fibrous network is in part responsible for the unique properties of articular cartilage, the physiological mechanisms that establish and maintain the orientation of individual collagen fibers are relatively unknown.

Hypotheses on the control of collagen fibril orientation have been approached from two separate disciplines: biological and biomechanical.

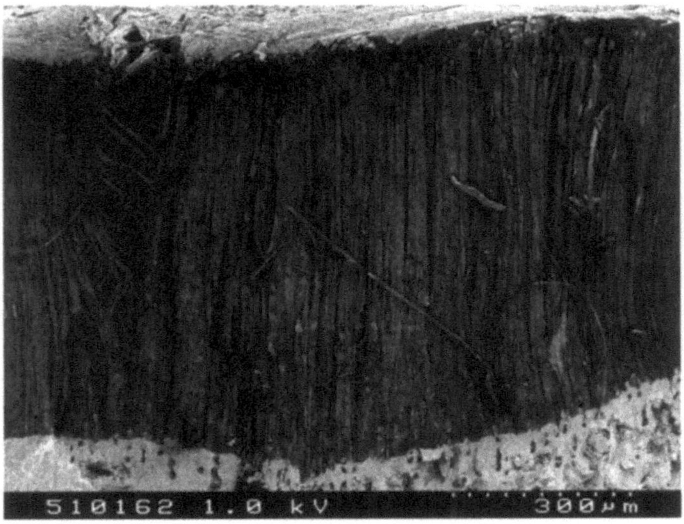

Fig. 3. Low magnification scanning electron micrograph of microwave-enhanced chemically fixed, and freeze-fractured rabbit medial tibial plateau cartilage with subchondral bone [from Richards (1996)]

The typical biological view is centered on the cell. Birk and Trelstad (1986, 1989) have presented morphological evidence for cellular control of fibril orientation in chick embryo cornea. They contend that collagen fibrils are formed within small cellular surface recesses that laterally fuse with other recesses to form collagen lamellae and bundles, thereby determining the architecture of the collagen network. However, no mechanistic evidence has been correlated with their morphological interpretations. Although their theory is plausible for the organization of the extracellular matrix near the cells (pericellular matrix) and in cellularly dense tissue, such as developing cornea, it is difficult to envision the means by which chondrocytes could orient fibrils in cartilage extracellular matrix. This matrix is so sparsely populated by cells and experiences repetitive deformation of its solid network and flow of its interstitial fluid.

In biomechanics, the prevalent approach has been that cartilage is optimal and the task is to find the criteria of optimality that will match the morphological attributes of the extracellular matrix. The investigations to date have shown that this optimal criteria may act through the physical environment of the extracellular matrix. Pauwels and his collaborators (1980) contend that collagen orientation in cartilage reflects its role as the tension resisting element. Split-line patterns (splits, produced by puncturing with a rounded awl, reflecting the tangential orientation of the collagen fibers in the STZ) from glenoid cavity cartilage specimens were correlated to the stress patterns from photoelastic gels with corresponding geometrical defects. Although no mechanisms were presented, they suggest that tension in the extracellular matrix per se orients the collagen.

Observations from other investigations also indicate that the collagen fiber architecture may be controlled by the physical environment of the extracellular matrix. Stopak et al. (1985), using a developing chicken limb bud model, concluded that forces exist within embryonic tissues that can arrange extracellular matrices into anatomical patterns. Fluorescent labeled type I collagen fibrils digested from rat tail tendons were injected near the developing shaft of a long bone. By confronting the embryo with pre-formed collagen fibrils, the biological mechanisms occurring during collagen deposition were avoided, yet these exogenous fibrils were found properly incorporated within the normal connective tissues of the developed wing. O'Conner et al. (1980) found that split-lines on the rat femoral condyles are well-defined only in the major load-bearing areas of the articular surface. Tepic (1982), comparing the femoral head of a newborn calf to that of a mature cow, found that these split-lines develop postnatally. Also, both Woo (1976) and Roth (1980) report isotropic tensile properties (reflecting an ordered collagen fibrillar architecture) as much more isotropic in skeletally immature compared to mature cartilage. The work of Tepic, Roth and Woo all indicate that collagen orientation develops during the postnatal growth period, and before skeletal maturity. Assuming smaller joint loads in utero, these observations are all consistent with the hypothesis that collagen orientation in cartilage is driven by forces generated within the extracellular matrix by physiological joint loads. In contrast to the solid stress-based hypothesis (tensile trajectories), we consider the poroelastic nature of cartilage, and postulate that collagen fiber network architecture is produced by interstitial fluid movement accompanying cartilage deformation during normal joint loading.

Movement-Induced Orientation Mechanism

Our movement-induced orientation proposal for collagen fibrils is motivated by the fact that short fibers can be oriented by movement relative to a finer, reticulated, three-dimensional, isotropic network (Laurent et al. 1975; Ogston et al. 1973). Such networks typically exist in gels. A true gel is a colloidal system, in which the network junctions are of infinite duration, giving the gel a non-zero equilibrium shear modulus. However, the orientation mechanism proposed herein is also compatible with a wider class of gel-like substances exemplified by entangled three-dimensional networks of polymer chains (Laurent et al. 1975).

The force acting on, and the resulting movement of, a fiber through an elastic/viscous medium is illustrated in Fig. 4. The elastic network of the medium is depicted by its nodes. Force F is the resultant body force on the fiber, inclined from the normal to the fiber by an angle α – components of F normal and parallel to the fiber are denoted as F_n and F_t, respectively. Force F_n is balanced by elastic stresses in the network. If F_t exceeds the piercing force F_p, the fiber moves, driven by the force $F_t - F_p$. As the fiber advances into a less strained area of the network the balance of forces is disturbed. Movement of the fiber out of the strained network at the rear, and its threading into a less strained network at the front, produces a net moment, tilting the fiber, as indicated by its next few positions in Fig. 4. The components F_n and F_t change as well: F_n decreasing, F_t increasing. The fiber turns and accelerates until the piercing force F_p and the viscous drag, induced in the fluid, balance the force F_t (ultimately F). The fiber then continues moving at a constant speed, oriented parallel to its trajectory (and force F).

After extracellular assembly and prior to incorporation into the extant collagen network, the new collagen fibrils are dispersed within a gel-like medium, the ubiquitous proteoglycans that form an entangled, molecular scale network of the extracellular matrix. The force to move the fibrils may be generated by the viscous drag of the fluid moving through the molecular (PG) network already immobilized by the extant collagen network. This fluid flow is created by the activities of daily living imposed

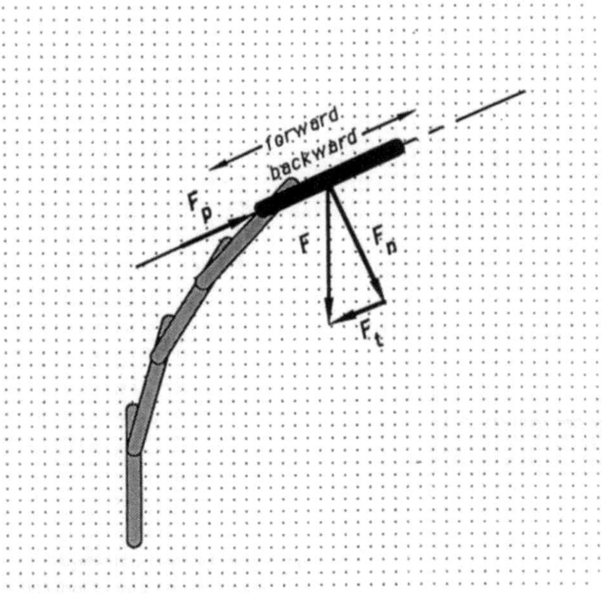

Fig. 4. Progression of a fiber (*F*) driven by forces through a poroelastic medium

on the tissue. Thus, the conditions of fibril movement through the fine, three-dimensional, PG network, we believe, give rise to orientation in the process of assembly of the coarse collagen network. However, for the proposed mechanism to function in cartilage, various conditions pertaining to the geometry and mechanical properties of the loose collagen fibrils and the PG network must be satisfied.

Movement-Induced Orientation Model

To evaluate this mechanism in cartilage, a simple model was developed incorporating the physical relationships required for this mechanism. In the model, the elastic portion of the network is represented as n elastic elements each with stress, σ_i, supporting the fiber with a lumped or body force, F, at the fiber centroid (Fig. 5a). The stress state of the network not directly underneath the fiber (but near the ends) is neglected, in a manner similar to the analysis of beams on an elastic foundation. The dissipative resistance or time-dependent motion, both perpendicular and parallel to the fiber axis, is represented with lumped elements. This resistance is the combination of the viscous resistance of: (1) the fluid on the fiber, (2) the fiber on the network, and (3) the network on the fluid (retardation of the network), where some or all of the above are applicable.

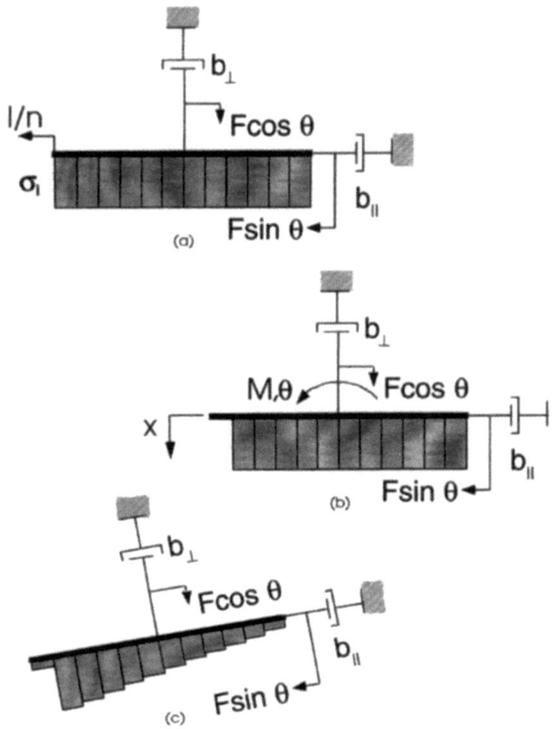

Fig. 5 a–c. Discreet time-dependent model of movement-induced orientation: **a** initial equilibrium, **b** after || movement l/n producing moment M, **c** re-establishment of equilibrium after time $dt = l\ b_{||}/n\ F \sin\theta$

The relaxation of the network is neglected, because for the step-loads used in the analysis, an elastically deformed part of the network always supports the fiber moving much like a pressure wave with the fiber. Damping coefficients are incorporated into the model as the resistance in the parallel direction (with respect to the fiber axis), $b_{||}$, and the ratio of this resistance to that in the perpendicular direction, $b_{\perp}/b_{||}$. Finally, the fiber of length, l, is assumed to be mass-less and rigid, with a diameter not much larger than the average pore size of the network. Hence, the elastic resistance of the network parallel to the fiber can be neglected.

The orienting moment, arising from the disturbance of the elastic restoring force of the network perpendicular to the fiber, is modeled in a discrete fashion. As the fiber moves forward by l/n, the energy stored in the elastic element no longer loaded by the fiber (the nth) is dissipated and the tip of the fiber moves into an unstrained network at the front (Fig. 5b). This imbalance of supporting force, $\Sigma\sigma_i$, and applied force, $F_n = F \cos\theta$, creates a moment, M, which causes the fiber to turn and translate perpendicularly in order to re-establish equilibrium (Fig. 5c). As the fiber proceeds to move by l/n along its axis, it continues to turn until it is parallel with the direction of the lumped or body force.

The model was validated by comparison to an analytical solution of a slender body sedimenting in a viscous fluid, and by experimental data of a fiber sedimenting in a 1% gelatin gel. For simulation of the viscous fluid, the network was made infinitely stiff (unable to store elastic energy) and the ratio of resistance perpendicular to the resistance parallel was set to 2.0 (Happel and Brenner 1983). The model predicts that the fiber does not turn and that the angle of the path is 19.5° to the vertical. This result is identical to the analytical solution for low Reynolds number flows (Happel and Brenner 1983). For validation against a physical model, the sedimentation of a stainless steel fiber in a 1% gelatin gel was recorded and digitized. The driving force was the measured weight of the fiber and the resistance in the parallel direction was calculated from the terminal velocity. Best fit values for network stiffness and $b_{\perp}$ were found using a modified feasible directions algorithm and least squares criterion (Vanderplaats 1984). The model-predicted path corresponded quite well to the gelatin experiment (Fig. 6). Hence, it can be concluded that this model has the basic physical relationships necessary to simulate the movement-induced mechanism in gel-like media for a wide variety of media ranging from a viscous fluid to a true gel.

Collagen in Cartilage Extracellular Matrix

To evaluate the potential of the movement-induced orientation mechanism for collagen in cartilage extracellular matrix, the parameter values

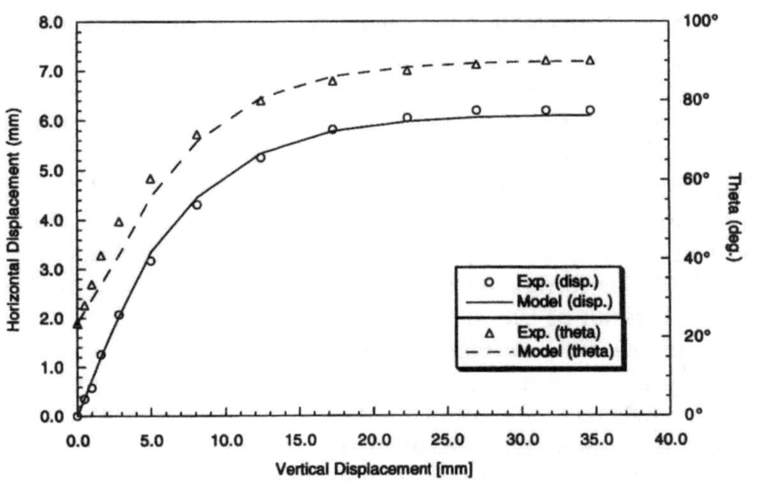

Fig. 6. Model-simulated path of a ∅ 0.6×12.6 mm stainless steel fiber sedimenting in a 1% gelatin solution

of collagen and cartilage extracellular matrix are required. Although they have not been directly measured it was possible to estimate them from known parameter values of the individual extracellular matrix components.

The drag force was calculated from fluid velocities and fibril geometry using potential fluid flow theory. The geometry of loose collagen fibrils, $\varnothing 10.4 \pm 0.5$ nm $\times$ 1.06 ± 0.03 μm, were taken from those isolated by irrigation of PG digested full-term bovine fetal femoral articular cartilage (patellar groove) (Ito 1994). The fluid velocity was calculated from joint consolidation and pressure measurements. Because the fluid is incompressible, the velocity of the fluid with respect to the solid matrix is approximately the rate of deformation of the joint surface. From the radiographic joint consolidation measurements of Armstrong et al. (1979) on loaded human cadaveric hip joints, the fluid velocity calculated from early creep is on the order of 1 μm/s. Using the formula for drag forces on a finite cylinder derived by Cox (1970), the drag force on the loose collagen fibrils is expressed as a function of the angle, θ between the fibril axis and the fluid flow. For $\theta = 90°$, the $F_{\perp} = 2.29 \times 10^{-15}$ N for a $\varnothing 10$ nm $\times$ 1 μm fibril.

After calculation of the drag force, the assumptions of a rigid massless fiber were verified. Assuming a simple, end-supported, cylindrical beam loaded with a lumped mid-beam force, equivalent to the drag force, the maximum deflection is only 0.69% of the fiber radius for a type I collagen with modulus of 1.4 GPa (Baer et al. 1988). With a molecular weight of 90 kDa for type II collagen molecules, the mass of the loose collagen fibril is approximately 22.1×10^{-21} kg, assuming 100% collagen per fibril. Since the accelerations in the model are less than 2×10^{-10} m/s^2, the inertial force experienced by the fiber is 10^{-15} of the drag force. Hence, our assumption of a rigid mass-less fiber was justified.

The stiffness of the PG network embedded within the extant collagen network was calculated from viscoelastic measurements of PG solutions and finite element analysis. As the loose collagen fibril is dragged by the fluid flow, it is forced to move relative to the fine molecular network of PGs. Hence, the stiffness of the network is that of the entangled PG molecule solution embedded in or fixed by the extant collagen network. The modulus for this PG network is different to that of cartilage. The modulus of cartilage is a result of Donnan osmotic equilibrium with bulk compression and exudative flow of interstitial fluid, whereas very little interstitial fluid is displaced and no bulk compression of the PG network occurs during the movement of the fibril. Using the viscoelastic measurements conducted by Mow et al. (1984b) on PG solutions of near physiological concentration and percent aggregation, the modulus of a physiological concentration (50 mg/ml) PG aggregate solution, assuming a Poisson's ratio of 0.5 (Mow et al. 1984b), is 5.6 Pa. This modulus was then used in a finite element model of the PG entangled network imbedded in the extant collagen network, created using geometry measured from transmission electron microscopy of the unloaded cartilage extracellular matrix (Ito 1994). Finally from the finite element model, a stiffness of 2.5×10^{-6} N/m was calculated for the PG aggregate entangled network embedded within the extant collagen network.

The dissipative resistance of the PG network to fibril motion may be due to two different modalities. In the first modality, the fibril moves through an entangled solution of PG aggregates with bulk flow of the PGs. In this case the dissipative resistance would simply be a function of the PG aggregate solution viscosity. In the second modality, the fibril moves through the entangled network of PG aggregates, but the PGs are bound at discreet points to the extant collagen network and experience no bulk motion. In the latter case the dissipative resistance would be due to the retardation of the network (dissipative resistance between the network and the interstitial water). Because the PG inter-monomer space on a hyaluronate backbone is similar to the loose collagen fibril diameter, the fibril probably displaces the individual PG monomers and deforms the PG aggregates, but would not displace PG aggregates relative to each other (Fig. 7). Hence, the dissipative resistance parallel to the fibril axis is probably the second modality and perpendicular to the fibril axis is the first modality. However, to distinguish between these two modalities may be too detailed considering the other assumptions in this analysis. Hence, the more demanding of the two modalities, the viscosity derived dissipative resistance, was used for further analysis. Because the PG aggregate

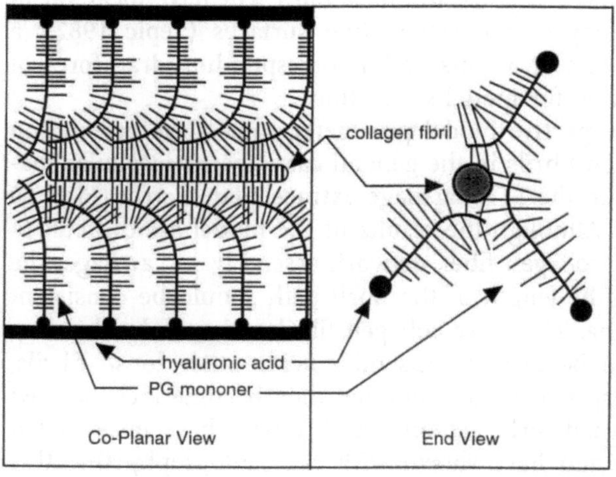

Fig. 7. A loose collagen fibril moving parallel to the fibril axis through the entangled PG network embedded in the extant collagen network

solution is a non-Newtonian fluid and has a shear rate dependent viscosity, the upper limit of the damping coefficients, $b_{\parallel}=3.64\times10^{-6}$ N s/m and $b_{\perp}/b_{\parallel}=1.64$, were calculated from the zero shear rate viscosity measured by Mow et al. (1984 a) for a 50 mg/ml PG aggregate solution.

Because of its unique extracellular matrix properties and the higher deformations, with regard to the deeper zones, the parameter values for the STZ were calculated separately. In this zone, Maroudas (1969) has shown, via the fixed charged density, that the glycosaminoglycan content is 40% of that found in the middle zone giving a PG aggregate concentration of approximately 20 mg/ml. From the viscoelastic measurements of Mow et al. (1984 b), this lower PG concentration corresponds to a lower elastic modulus of 1.04 Pa for the PG network and a stiffness of 0.46×10^{-6} N/m for the entangled PG aggregate network embedded in the extant collagen network. Also, with a lower PG concentration, the zero shear rate viscosity becomes 0.5 N s/m^2 and the corresponding $b_{\parallel}$ is 7.0×10^{-7} N s/m for the dissipative resistance to fibril motion.

In addition to these different PG network characteristics, the interstitial fluid velocity is higher in this zone. If we examine a cylindrical control volume into the depth of cartilage, the fluid expressed during consolidation must flow either tangentially through the cartilage or out and through the interarticular gap. Macirowski (1994) showed the conductance of the interarticular gap in the hip is less than one third of the conductance through the tissue. Hence, two thirds of the expressed fluid flows tangentially through the STZ. With a surface displacement rate 1 μm/s (Armstrong et al. 1979), contact area radius of 10 mm in the acetabulum (Tepic 1982) and an STZ depth of 100 μm (Meachim and Stockwell 1979), the tangential average velocity in the human hip joint is approximately 30 μm/s. However, since the flow rates will have local variations due to incongruency of the articulating surfaces (Tepic 1982), a more conservative flow rate of 5 μm/s and a corresponding drag force of $F_{\perp}=1.15\times10^{-14}$ N was used for model simulations.

Finally, using these respective model parameter values, the orientation and path of loose collagen fibrils in the general cartilage extracellular matrix (Figs. 8 and 9) and in the STZ cartilage extracellular matrix (Figs. 10 and 11) were simulated. Although the results of the model are difficult to evaluate with respect to collagen fiber network assembly in cartilage, the time to orientation and the length of the fibril path should be consistent with observed phenomena. The loose collagen fibrils oriented by the drag induced mechanism are believed to assemble with other loose fibrils, after orientation, into larger banded fibers that then become incorporated into the extant collagen network. Leblond et al. (1981) have investigated this incorporation rate, and have shown with radioautography that this occurs within one to several days for dentin and bone matrix. Assuming that the rate of collagen fibril incorporation into the extant network for

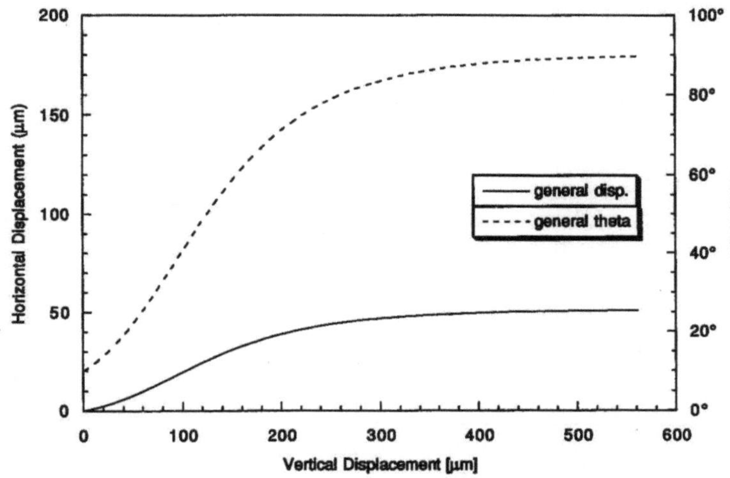

Fig. 8. Model-predicted path of the loose collagen fibril in cartilage extracellular matrix

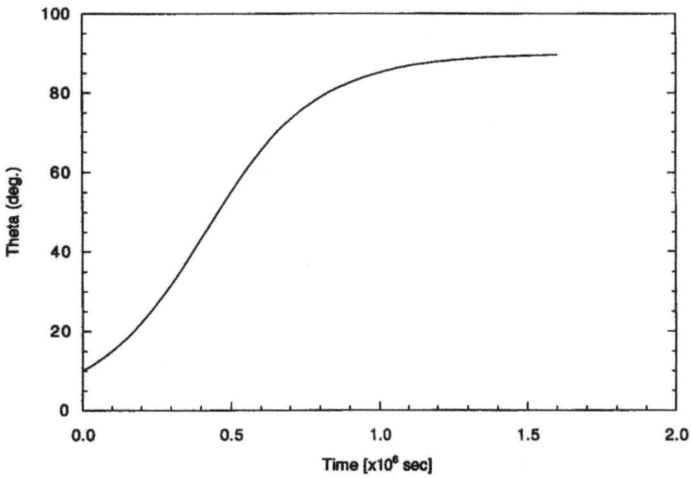

Fig. 9. Model-predicted orientation of the loose collagen fibril in cartilage extracellular matrix

cartilage is of a similar order of magnitude to that of bone, under physiological loading conditions, the mechanism must orient the loose collagen fibrils within days. In the general cartilage matrix, the model predicts that the loose collagen fibril would require more than 2 weeks for orientation under similar conditions, but in the special case of the STZ, the model predicts that loose collagen fibrils will become oriented within an hour. Thus, this model supports the movement-induced orientation mechanism hypothesis only within the STZ of cartilage.

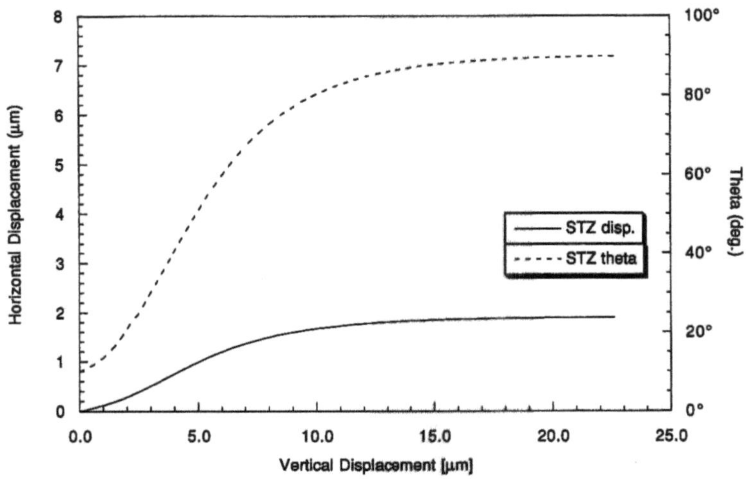

Fig. 10. Model-predicted path of the loose collagen fibril in the superficial tangential zone of cartilage extracellular matrix

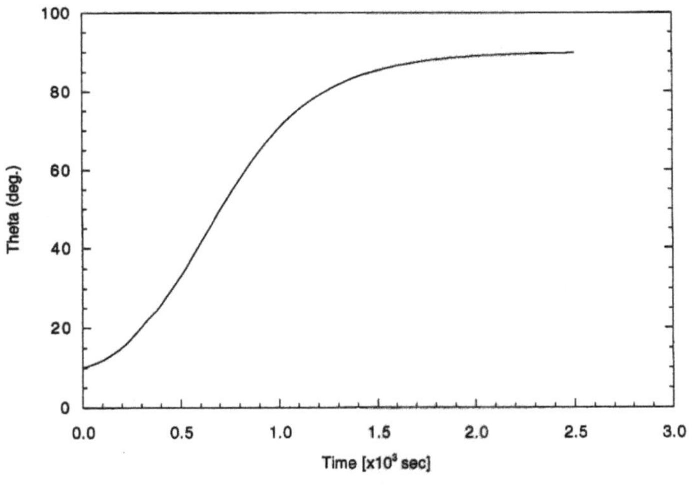

Fig. 11. Model-predicted orientation of the loose collagen fibril in the superficial tangential zone of cartilage extracellular matrix

With respect to the fibril path length, its rather extreme length is a result of the constant drag force used to drive the model. Under a step load, the predicted translational movement of the fibril can be up to 600 µm for flow rates of 1 µm/s (Fig. 8) and 23 µm for flow rates of 5 µm/s in the STZ (Fig. 10). However, under the activities of daily life, articular cartilage is subjected to cyclical loads, and hence the fluid flows and drag forces are also cyclical. Although a cyclically loaded model was not simulated, characteristics of the cyclical response can be inferred from the step load response. First, under cyclical loading the fibril would not travel such great distances but would be dragged to and fro, gradually orienting, but not translating significantly. Of course, the average intensity of the flow would also be decreased with cyclical loads and the orientation would require more time, but for sinusoidal flow cycles, the intensity would only decrease by one half, and the fibril would still become oriented within 24 h. Finally, in the above model, relaxation of the PG network was neglected because a portion of the network directly under the fibril is always elastically deformed. However, with decreased frequency of cyclical motion, the PG network will relax, with some loss of the elastic stored energy. This change in the elastic nature of the PG network with frequency was included in the model by calculating the elasticity of the PG network at 1 Hz, the physiological loading rate. Hence, under the more physiological conditions of cyclical load, the model results indicate that the movement-induced orientation mechanism has the potential to orient loose collagen fibrils in the superficial zones of articular cartilage. In the deeper zones of articular cartilage, the flow velocity does not appear sufficient for such an orientation mechanism to function, and the radial orientation of the large fibers observed in this zone may be a result of tissue growth.

Significance

Animal studies have suggested that joint loading and motion can elicit various biological responses in articular cartilage. Immobilization has been found to decrease PG synthesis and content (Caterson and Lowther 1978) resulting in tissue softening (Jurvelin et al. 1989). In the major load-bearing areas of cartilage, the PG content is often higher (Slowman and Brandt 1986), and can even be increased by more dynamic loading (Caterson and Lowther 1978). Furthermore, remobilization of an immobilized joint can often return to normal the PG synthesis rates and content levels (Jurvelin et al. 1989).

The qualitative results seen in these animal studies have been confirmed and quantified using explant models. It has been shown that while static compression significantly inhibits PG and protein synthesis, dynamic compression can stimulate matrix production (Sah et al. 1989). This biological response to loading may be modulated by various physical phenomenon in the cartilage, e.g. osmotic pressure, fixed charged density, cell deformation, streaming potentials, pressure gradients, fluid flows, etc. However, the experiments of Kim et al. (1995) indicate that fluid flow phenomenon is currently the most consistent with observations. They compressed cartilage discs between two non-porous plattens to produce non-uniform spatial profiles of fluid velocity. At higher frequencies, hydrostatic pressure was highest in the center of these discs, whereas fluid velocities were greatest at the periphery. The observed synthetic patterns most closely matched the radial distribution of fluid flow. Thus, the stimulation of chondrocyte matrix synthesis by dynamic load appears to be through the mechanism of fluid flow, similar to the organization mechanism of the collagen network architecture.

If indeed articular cartilage matrix synthesis and collagen architecture is dependent on joint loading and fluid flow, what are the clinical implications? With the demonstration of the limited regeneration capacity of native articular cartilage, engineered tissue substitutes and autografts have been advocated as biological replacement material. Although the morphologies of these replacements may be similar to that of the native cartilage, their biomechanical properties are often insufficient. It has already been recognized that dynamic loading during engineered tissue growth may enhance extracellular matrix synthesis and chondrocyte proliferation rates. In addition, dynamic loading of engineered cartilage may be required to generate native like collagen fiber architectures. Ultimately, for the long-term survival and performance of any cartilage replacement, joint loading and particularly interstitial fluid flow may be necessary.

Conclusion

Articular cartilage provides a durable, low-friction, load-bearing surface for our synovial joints. This performance results in part from a well-organized collagen fiber network architecture. Teleological arguments have dominated past interpretations of cartilage structure (Pauwels 1980; Roux 1985) leaving the collagen orientation mechanism unresolved.

All connective tissues are poroelastic and their loading results in both deformation and fluid flow. We postulate that collagen orientation is induced by fluid movement, whereby newly assembled, yet unlinked, stiff collagen fibrils are dragged through the extracellular matrix (Tepic and Ito 1997). Fibril orientation arises through its elastic interaction with the molecular-scale network of proteoglycans found in the extracellular matrix. Collagen architecture is the result of cross-linking these oriented fibrils into the extant collagen network.

This movement-induced orientation mechanism has already been demonstrated for movement of DNA segments in hyaluronate solutions (Laurent et al. 1975). Most recently, a simulation model has been developed for this orientation mechanism (Ito et al. 1999). With physiological parameter values, it has demonstrated the potential of movement-induced collagen fibril orientation in articular cartilage.

With recent developments in tissue engineering for treatment of damaged cartilage, the effect of loading on cartilage has become clinically relevant. It has been recognized that dynamic loading of cartilage enhances extracellular matrix synthesis and chondrocyte proliferation rates (Grodzinski et al. 1998). Furthermore, dynamic loading of engineered cartilage may be required to generate native-like collagen network architectures important for biomechanical performance.

Acknowledgment. This work was supported in part by a grant from the AO ASIF Foundation.

References

Armstrong CG, Bahrani AS, Gardner MA (1979) In vitro measurement of articular cartilage deformations in the intact human hip joint under load. J Bone Joint Surg 61A:744–755

Baer E, Cassidy JJ, Hiltner A (1988) Hierarchical structure of collagen and its relationship to the physical properties of tendon. In: Nimni ME (ed) Collagen CRC Press Inc., Boca Raton, pp 177–199

Benninghoff A (1925) Form und Bau der Gelenkknorpel in ihren Beziehungen zur Funktion. Z Zellforsch 2:783–862

Birk DE, Trelstad RL (1986) Extracellular compartments in tendon morphogenesis: collagen fibril, bundle, and macroaggregate formation. J Cell Biol 103:231–240

Birk DE, Zycband EI, Winkelmann DA, Trelstad RL (1989) Collagen fibrillogenesis in situ: fibril segments are intermediates in matrix assembly. Proc Natl Acad Sci USA 86:4549–4553

Bowden FP, Tabor D (1950) The friction and lubrication of solids. Oxford University Press, London, pp 165–166

Caterson B, Lowther DA (1978) Changes in the metabolism of the proteoglycans from sheep articular cartilage in response to mechanical stress. Biochim Biophys Acta 540:412–422

Charnley J (1959) Lubrication of animal joints. Inst Mech Eng, London, Proc Symp Biomech, pp 12–22

Clark JM (1985) The organization of collagen in cryofractured rabbit articular cartilage: a scanning electron microscopic study. J Orthop Res 3:17–29

Cox RG (1970) The motion of long slender bodies in a viscous fluid part I: general theory. J Fluid Mech 44:791–810

Grodzinsky AJ, Kim YJ, Buschmann MD, Garcia AM, Quinn TM, Hunziker EB (1998) Response of the chondrocyte to mechanical stimuli. In: Brandt KD, Doherty M, Lohmander LS (eds) Osteoarthritis. Oxford University Press, New York, pp 123–136

Happel J, Brenner H (1983) Low Reynolds number hydrodynamics. Martinus Nijhoff, Den Hague

Ito K (1994) Movement-induced orientation of collagen fibrils in cartilaginous tissues (ScD Thesis). Massachusetts Institute of Technology, Cambridge, Massachusetts

Ito K, Tepic S, Mann RW (1996) A mechanism for the orientation of collagen in cartilage. 42nd Annual Meeting of the Orthopaedic Research Society, Atlanta, Georgia, 21:568

Jones ES (1936) Joint lubrication. Lancet 1:1043–1044

Jurvelin J, Kiviranta I, Saamanen AM, Tammi M, Helminen HJ (1989) Partial restoration of immobilization-induced softening of canine articular cartilage after remobilization of the knee (stifle) joint. J Orthop Res 7:352–358

Kääb MJ, Richards RG, Nötzli H (1996) Microwave enhanced preservation for morphologic studies of articular cartilage. 42nd Annual Meeting of the Orthopaedic Research Society. Orthopaedic Research Society 21:323

Kim YJ, Bonassar LJ, Grodzinsky AJ (1995) The role of cartilage streaming potential, fluid flow and pressure in the stimulation of chondrocyte biosynthesis during dynamic compression. J Biomech 28:1055–1066

Laurent TC, Preston BN, Pertoft H, Gustaffson B, McCabe M (1975) Diffusion of linear polymers in hyaluronate solutions. Eur J Biochem 53:129–136

LeBlond CP, Wright GM (1981) Steps in the elaboration of collagen by odontoblasts and osteoblasts. In: Hand AR, Oliver C (eds) Methods in cell biology. Academic Press, New York, pp 167–189

Macirowski T, Tepic S, Mann RW (1994) Cartilage stresses in the human hip joint. J Biomech Eng 116:10–18

Maroudas A (1979) Physicochemical properties of articular cartilage. In: Freeman MAR (ed) Adult articular cartilage. Pitman Medical, Tunbridge Wells, Kent, pp 215–290

Maroudas A, Muir H, Wingham J (1969) The correlation of fixed negative charge with glycosaminoglycan content of human articular cartilage. Biochim Biophys Acta 177:492–500

Meachim G, Stockwell RA (1979) The matrix. In: Freeman MAR (ed) Adult articular cartilage. Pitman Medical, Tunbridge Wells, Kent, pp 1–50

Mow VC, Holmes MH, Lai WM (1984a) Fluid transport and mechanical properties of articular cartilage: a review. J Biomech 17:377–394

Mow VC, Mak AF, Lai WM (1984b) Viscoelastic properties of proteoglycan subunits and aggregates in varying solution concentrations. J Biomech 17:325–338

Nimni ME (1975) Molecular structure and function of collagen in normal and diseased tissues. In: Burleigh PM, Poole AR (eds) Dynamics of connective tissue macromolecules. American Elsevier, New York, pp 33–79

O'Conner P, Bland C, Gardner DL (1980) Fine structure of artificial splits in femoral condylar cartilage of the rat: a scanning electron microscopic study. J Path 132: 169–179

Ogston AG, Preston BN, Wells JD (1973) On the transport of compact particles through solutions of chain polymers. Proc Royal Soc (London) A333:297–309

Orkin RW, Pratt RM, Martin GR (1976) Undersulfated chondroitin sulfate in the cartilage matrix of brachymorphic mice. Develop Biol 50:82–94

Pauwels F (1980) Biomechanics of the locomotor apparatus. Springer, Berlin Heidelberg New York

Richards RG, Kääb MJ (1996) Microwave-enhanced fixation of rabbit articular cartilage. J Microscopy 181:269–276

Roth V, Mow VC (1980) The intrinsic tensile behavior of the matrix of bovine articular cartilage and its variation with age. J Bone Joint Surg 62:1102–1117

Roux W (1985) Beitrag für Morphologie der funktionellen Anpassung. 3. Beschreibung und Erläuterung einer knöchernen Kniegelenksankylose. Archiv Anat Phys Wissensch Med, pp 120–158

Sah RL, Kim YJ, Doong JY, Grodzinsky AJ, Plaas AH, Sandy JD (1989) Biosynthetic response of cartilage explants to dynamic compression. J Orthop Res 7:619–636

Slowman SD, Brandt KD (1986) Composition and glycosaminoglycan metabolism of articular cartilage from habitually loaded and habitually unloaded sites. Arthritis Rheum 29:88–94

Stopak D, Wessells NK, Harris AK (1985) Morphogenetic rearrangement of injected collagen in developing chicken limb buds. Proc Natl Acad Sci USA 82:2804–2808
Tepic S (1982) Dynamics of and entropy production in the cartilage layers of the synovial joint (ScD Thesis). Massachusetts Institute of Technology, Cambridge, Massachusetts
Tepic S, Ito K (1997) Orientation mechanisms of collagen. In: Schneider E (ed) Biomechanik des menschlichen Bewegungsapparates. Springer, Berlin Heidelberg New York, pp 204–214
Vanderplaats GN (1984) Numerical optimization techniques for engineering design: with applications. McGraw-Hill, New York
Venn M, Maroudas A (1977) Chemical composition of normal and osteoarthrotic femoral head cartilage. Ann Rheum Dis 36:121–129
Weiss C, Rosenberg L, Helfet AJ (1968) An ultrastructural study of normal young adult human articular cartilage. J Bone Joint Surg [Am] 50:663–674
Woo SLY, Akeson WH, Jemmott GF (1976) Measurement of nonhomogeneous directional mechanical properties of articular cartilage in tension. J Biomech 9:785–791

Pharmacological Basis for the Therapy of Osteoarthritis

J. Steinmeyer

Introduction

For a targeted pharmacologically oriented basic therapy for osteoarthritis, it is important that the drugs should act against the underlying process of cartilage destruction. A deep insight and exact knowledge of the pathogenetic reactions that occur during the course of degenerative joint disease are necessary for the development of such agents. Fortunately, from the field of experimental osteoarthritis research, a large number of new and interesting findings have come to light over the last 5–10 years concerning the pathogenesis of osteoarthritic joint dysfunction. In order to illustrate the present possible starting points for a pharmacological intervention, some aspects of the pathogenesis of osteoarthritis is first briefly described as it is currently understood.

Special Aspects in Pathogenesis

In healthy articular cartilage an equilibrium exists between the anabolic and catabolic activities of the chondrocytes. In osteoarthritic joints, a disturbance in this equilibrium occurs, which ultimately leads to a degradation and loss of cartilaginous tissue. The essential pathophysiological changes within osteoarthritic joint cartilage that lead to a progressive destruction of that tissue include the increased breakdown of type II collagen and proteoglycans (Mankin and Brandt 1997). Previous studies concentrated primarily upon the destruction of aggrecan and collagen, although proteolytic destruction of other molecules such as link proteins, fibronectin, decorin, etc., might also fatally influence the integrity of articular cartilage. Histological and biochemical studies show that the destruction of the collagen fibers occurs with an increased biosynthesis of collagenases, enzymes that belong to the matrix-metalloproteinase (MMP) family. Biochemical analysis of the proteoglycan fragments revealed that a proteolytic breakdown of proteoglycans occurs in vivo. The proteoglycans can be broken down by various MMPs (e.g. stromelysin), as well as other proteases (e.g. plasmin, aggrecanase, PMN elastase)

(Nagase and Okada 1997; Sandy et al. 1992). The activity of these MMPs is controlled by endogenously occurring inhibitors, known as tissue inhibitors of metalloproteinases (TIMP), which are also synthesized by the chondrocytes (Nagase and Okada 1997).

MMPs such as stromelysin and collagenase are secreted as proenzymes and have to be activated extracellularly in a multi-step process before they can cleave their substrates (Nagase and Okada 1997). Figure 1 summarizes the present knowledge and hypotheses concerning the biosynthesis, activation and activity of MMPs and their role in the destruction of articular cartilage (Mankin and Brandt 1997; Nagase and Okada 1997; Pelletier and Martel-Pelletier 1993; Pelletier and Howell 1993): within this scheme, the serine protease plasmin is partly involved in the activation of MMPs. Plasmin is produced from plasminogen as a result of the activity of plasminogen activators (tPA; uPA). The activity of these serine proteases is in turn regulated by the PAI-1 (plasminogen activator inhibitor-1) content of the tissue. Interestingly, there is not only an increased biosynthesis of these plasminogen activators in osteoarthritic articular cartilage, but there is also a drastically reduced content of PAI-1; as a result of both these processes, an increased formation of plasmin from plasminogen occurs. Plasmin in turn activates the latently occurring MMPs,

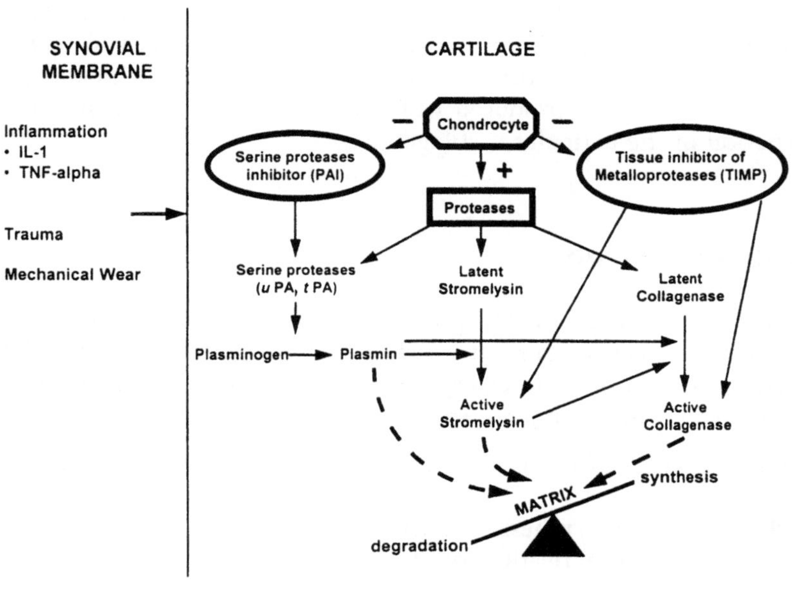

Fig. 1. Some major factors involved in catabolism of articular cartilage [modified from Pelletier and Howell (1993)]. Note that stromelysin and collagenase are mentioned as examples of important matrix-metalloproteinases (MMPs) involved in catabolism of cartilage. *IL-1*, interleukin-1; *TNF-alpha*, tumor necrosis factor-alpha

which then degrade the extracellular matrix of the articular cartilage. With the increasing destruction of the articular cartilage, fragments of collagen, proteoglycans and possibly other extracellular matrix components can gain access to the synovial fluid where they can induce or exacerbate inflammatory reactions. The inflammation is more than likely responsible for the increased levels of interleukin-1 (IL-1), which are often measured in the synovial fluid of osteoarthritic patients. The cytokine IL-1 influences the chondrocytes so that they produce more MMPs and plasminogen activators while the biosynthesis of important physiological inhibitors, such as TIMP-1 and PAI-1, are reduced. Furthermore, IL-1 acts to reduce the biosynthesis of collagen and proteoglycans. The imbalance between the levels of catabolic enzymes and their natural inhibitors leads to an increased content of active MMPs. This, combined with the reduced biosynthesis of extracellular matrix, results in a severe damage of the articular cartilage.

Although, (1) osteoarthritis has a multiple etiology and, (2) both mechanic and biochemical/metabolic factors play essential roles in this disease, one or more of the above-mentioned factors appear to be responsible for the increased content of proteolytic enzymes that are synthesized by the chondrocytes and that definitively take part in the progressive destruction of articular cartilage. As a consequence of this destruction there is an increased release of extracellular matrix fragments into the synovial fluid where they can bring about or exacerbate an inflammatory reaction of the synovial membrane. Inflammation of the synovial membrane leads to an increased formation of, for example, IL-1 with the effect that a vicious circle is produced which leads ultimately to a progressive destruction of the articular cartilage.

Pharmacological Concepts

The pathogenetic findings already presented allowed the development of a pharmaceutical strategy aimed at providing a specific basic therapy for osteoarthritis. As such, it is necessary to synthesize and/or validate drugs that are effective in the catabolic area:

1. As direct inhibitors of the catabolically active MMPs and aggrecanase and/or
2. As blockers of the biosynthesis of such catabolic enzymes, and/or
3. As inhibitors of the activation of precursor enzymes to their active forms, and/or
4. As stimulators of the biosynthesis of endogenously occurring inhibitors (TIMP-1, PAI-1) and/or,
5. As inhibitors of proinflammatory cytokines.

It also seems sensible and indeed desirable to develop agents that can increase the anabolic functions of chondrocytes concerning their ability to synthesize the extracellular matrix.

It can be expected from such agents that the proteolytic destruction of the articular cartilage would be stopped or at least decelerated so that the progression of osteoarthritis is counteracted.

Presently Available Medications

Apart from the fast-acting nonsteroidal antiinflammatory and analgesic drugs, a number of other well-tolerated and effective preparations are available for a medication-based symptomatic treatment of osteoarthritis; the latter have been termed by the Osteoarthritis Research Society (OARS 1992) as "slow acting drugs in osteoarthritis (OA)", or SADOAs for short (Bach 1996; Lequesne 1993). The term "chondroprotection" was coined in 1983 by Annefeld and Fassbender; this described the protective effects of individual nonsteroidal antiinflammatory drugs against ultrastructural changes induced in rat chondrocytes by massive doses of corticosteroids. This term is somewhat antiquated today and should no longer be used. Other drugs exist for which an antiarthritic effectiveness has been postulated and that have no defined mechanism of action (e.g. homeopathic agents, gelatin, various mixed preparations of organ extracts or lysates). According to the recommendations of the OARS, SADOAs can be classified concerning their effectiveness into the following subgroups:

1. Symptomatically effective preparations: symptomatic slow acting drugs in OA (SYSADOAs); included amongst these are ademethionine (GUMBARAL), D-glucosamine sulfate (DONA 200 S), oxaceprole (AHP-200), and hyaluronic acid (HYALART).
2. Disease modifying OA drugs (DMOADs). These, according to definition, inhibit, decelerate or even reverse morphologically definable cartilage defects in human clinical studies. For this property – with its activity directed towards hyaline cartilage – no clinical evidence has so far been provided since the validation of biochemical/immunological parameters or imaging procedures, for example, remains outstanding.

The recommendations of a group of international scientific arthritis societies concerning the standardized testing and registration requirements for osteoarthritis medications led in 1996 to a subclassification of drugs into groups of: (1) "symptom modifying drugs", and (2) "structure modifying drugs" with/without an additional antisymptomatic activity (Dougados 1996).

In the following, the most significant findings on the effects of SYSADOAs on articular cartilage that were determined in in vitro and animal experimental studies will be presented. It has to be stressed, however, that the presented mosaic of in vitro and animal in vivo studies cannot be extrapolated to the human clinical situation without reservations.

In Vitro Studies on Cell and/or Cartilage Explant Cultures

The influence of SYSADOAs on chondrocyte metabolism has been investigated by several research groups. Ademethionine ($\geq 10^{-6}$ M), D-glucosamine sulfate ($\geq 10^{-5}$ M), hyaluronic acid (1 mg/ml) and oxaceprole ($\geq 10^{-9}$ M) all stimulate the synthesis of proteoglycans by cultured chondrocytes obtained from various species (Bassleer et al. 1993; Harmand et al. 1987; Kalbhen and Kalkert 1987; Riera et al. 1990; Tanaka et al. 1997). In order to determine how far the results of in vitro experiments are therapeutically significant, one has to know the concentrations of the agents in the synovial fluid, or at least in patient serum, after a therapeutic dose is given. As such, Stramentinoli (1987) reported that the concentration of ademethionine in patients' synovial fluid after giving a therapeutic dose was in the order of 10^{-7} M. The concentrations of D-glucosamine sulfate or oxaceprole in patients' synovial fluid after therapeutic dosing, however, are not currently known. If one assumes similar sized molecules and similar dosing, it can be presumed that the concentration of each of the agents would also be around 10^{-7} M in the patients' synovial fluid. In man, therefore, the proteoglycan synthesis stimulating effect of ademethionine and D-glucosamine sulfate would only be brought about at concentrations in the synovial fluid between 10- and 100-fold higher than those that are actually achievable after an oral therapeutic dose. Animal experimental studies (Laurent et al. 1992; Engfeldt and Hjertquist 1967) show that the half life of hyaluronic acid in the joints is between 13 and 20 h, with the result that this medication is completely eliminated from the joints after 3–4 days. When one considers that a hyaluronic acid therapy is usually dosed in 5×20 mg intra-articular injections given at weekly intervals, this would mean that a stimulating effect on proteoglycan synthesis could only be expected during the first couple of days after injection.

The investigations by Vivien et al. (1993) are also interesting. They determined that $\geq 10^{-6}$ M oxaceprole not only stimulates collagen synthesis to a small extent in cultured human chondrocytes, but that it also inhibits the IL-1 induced release of collagen from rabbit articular cartilage. Here, it is certainly true that the concentrations used were somewhat higher compared to the presumed concentrations of this medication in patients' synovial fluid. On the other hand, Riera et al. (1990) reported that even high concentrations of oxaceprole could not inhibit the catabolic breakdown of proteoglycans and the accompanying loss of proteoglycans from bovine articular cartilage explants. In contrast, several studies have shown that hyaluronic acid even at low concentrations (0.1–1.5 mg/ml) can inhibit the IL-1-induced, tumor necrosis factor-alpha-induced or fibronectin fragment-induced loss of proteoglycans from articular cartilage explants obtained from various species (Akatsuka et al. 1993; Homandberg et al. 1997; Morris et al. 1992; Shimazu et al. 1993). This inhibitory effect on the cytokine-induced loss of proteoglycans may arise because the hyaluronic acid forms a film over the cartilage surface and thereby prevents the penetration of IL-1 TNF-alpha or fibronectin fragments. When considering the short half-life of hyaluronic acid within the joint, it is clear that such an effect could only be apparent for a few days.

Enzyme Kinetic Studies

As has already been mentioned, the inhibition of MMPs and/or aggrecanase activity can contribute significantly to an anticatabolic action. On this subject, several interesting studies have already been published. Hence, ademethionine and D-glucosamine sulfate, even at high concentrations (10^{-4} M), had no inhibitory effects on the activity of MMPs that partake in proteoglycan and collagen breakdown (Steinmeyer and Daufeldt 1997; Hübner et al. 1997). Ademethionine and oxaceprole also exert no inhibitory effects on the activity of plasmin or plasminogen activators that clearly take part, as already mentioned, in the activation of latent secreted MMPs (Steinmeyer at al. 1996).

Further studies will help to resolve whether these pharmaceuticals affect the biosynthesis of these catabolic enzymes or their natural inhibitors. One study has shown that D-glucosamine sulfate reduces the MMP stromelysin mRNA content in cultures of human chondrocytes at a high concentration of 5×10^{-6} M (Jiménez and Dodge 1997). However, it should be pointed out that a raised or reduced mRNA content does not allow any statement to be made concerning the quantities of newly formed molecules since the synthesized mRNA can be subjected to many types of post-translational modification. Hyaluronic acid has also been investigated for its effects on the biosynthesis of TIMP and stromelysin, whereby contradictory results have been reported; a reduced, unchanged or even increased biosynthesis of stromelysin has been described (Akatsuka et al. 1993; Homandberg et al. 1997; Yasui et al. 1992). Yasui et al. (1992) showed raised synthesis of both stromelysin and TIMP, whereby the ratio of TIMP to stromelysin was shifted in favor of the TIMP.

Animal Experimental Studies

The clinical evaluation of the intensity and progression of degenerative human joint disorders is presently still very difficult; this is because both the beginning and early symptom-free phase of the degeneration process cannot be determined exactly. Furthermore, no adequate, standardized parameters are available for a quantitative objective evaluation of advanced osteoarthritis. From an experimental point of view, and for ethical reasons, animal experiments offer the advantage that an objective evaluation parameter can be measured that describes the disease modifying effect on the articular cartilage. In other words, one can check whether the drug – at least in animal experiments – has a basic therapeutic effect, i.e. one that results in protection or even regeneration of the articular cartilage, since the joint can be investigated biochemically and histologically at the end of such experiments. Several animal experimental studies have been published on this matter.

In the model used by Kalbhen et al. (1987), Kalbhen and Jansen (1990), osteoarthritic changes in chicken knee joints were biochemically induced by injecting monoiodoacetic acid. Using this model, ademethionine (0.5–2 mg), D-glucosamine sulfate (0.02–12 mg), hyaluronic acid (0.01–1 mg), or oxaceprole (0.01–1 mg), injected intra-articularly 1–2 times weekly produced no significant reduction in the intensity or progression of degenerative changes in the chicken knee joints. In the same study, however, 1 mg ademethionine was found to be effective. Such a lack of a dose-dependent effect is unusual within the field of pharmacology and there is no explanation for it at the present time. It should also be mentioned, however, that when ademethionine, D-glucosamine sulfate and oxaceprole are dosed orally, substantially lower amounts of these drugs are found in the synovial fluid than are seen after intra-articular injection.

In another animal experimental study (Raiss 1985), a 24 mg intramuscularly injected dose of D-glucosamine sulfate given twice weekly provided a certain protective effect against dexamethasone-induced degenerative changes in rat articular cartilage.

Another in vivo model, in which osteoarthritic changes were induced mechanically by a partial meniscectomy, the effect of ademethionine and hyaluronic acid on articular cartilage of rabbits was investigated (Barcelo et al. 1987; Kikuchi et al. 1996). Ademethionine intra-muscular injections given daily over a period of 12 weeks (30 or 60 mg/kg per day) resulted in significant increases in both cartilage cell-counts and cartilage thickness (Barcelo et al. 1987). The increase in cartilage thickness allows us to presume that ademethionine has a stimulating effect on the anabolic functions of the chondrocytes. Hyaluronic acid (0.1 ml/kg, 10 mg/ml), injected intra-articularly twice weekly – which does not correspond to the human therapeutic dosing – reduced the histopathologically recognizable degeneration of articular cartilage (Kikuchi et al. 1996).

The effect of hyaluronic acid was also studied on experimental osteoarthritis in the rabbit knee which underwent unilateral anterior cruciate ligament transection (ACLT) (Yoshioka et al. 1997; Shimizu et al. 1998). 0.3 ml hyaluronan (ARTZ), having a molecular weight of 8×10^5, was intra-articularly injected once a week for 5 weeks beginning 4 weeks after ACLT. The contralateral nonoperated knee served as control. The morphologic, histomorphometric and biochemical results of these studies indicated that hyaluronan has a protective effect on the articular cartilage up to 21 weeks post-ACLT.

Hyaluronic acid was intensively investigated in Australia by Prof. Ghosh's group using a sheep model (Armstrong et al. 1994; Ghosh 1994; Ghosh et al. 1995). In this model, osteoarthritis in the knee joint was mechanically induced by a partial meniscectomy. The sheeps received hyaluronic acid (2 ml, 10 mg/ml) by intra-articular injection once weekly over a period of 5 weeks. Interestingly, a preparation consisting of 900 kDa hyaluronate reduced the histopathologically recognizable degeneration of articular cartilage, the rebuilding of the subchondral bone, and the loss of proteoglycans into the synovial fluid. Conversely, an increased formation of both osteophytes and cartilage lesions was seen after intra-articular application of a higher molecular weight hyaluronic acid preparation. The investigators presumed that the higher molecular weight hyaluronate preparation improved joint lubrication in such way that joint usage by the animals was intensified so that the osteoarthritic disease process was in fact accelerated.

Studies on Anti-inflammatory and Analgesic Effects

In a series of animal studies, ademethionine, D-glucosamine sulfate, hyaluronic acid and oxaceprole were all shown to have an anti-inflammatory effect while only ademethionine, hyaluronic acid and oxaceprole had also an analgesic effect (Gotoh et al. 1988; Gualano et al. 1985; Ialante and Di Rosa 1994; Ionac et al. 1996; Miyazaki et al. 1984; Setnikar et al. 1991a; Setnikar et al. 1991b; Weischer 1987). On the basis of these results, one of the indications for these drugs is activated osteoarthritis. The analgesic and anti-inflammatory effects do not result from an inhibition of prostaglandin synthesis, since no inhibitory effect on cyclooxygenases could be found. Hence, these drugs do not number among the classic nonsteroidal antiinflammatory drugs that are known to inhibit prostaglandin synthesis by inhibiting cyclooxygenases.

Clinical studies serving as evidence for the effectiveness of these drugs have usually quoted subjective observations such as freedom from pain or return of normal mobility as criteria for evaluating their effectiveness. These parameters, however, provide no information as to whether a progressive cartilage disruption in osteoarthritis is decelerated, stopped, and/or reversed. A series of clinical studies also exists in which the effects of SYSADOAs have been examined using the Lequesne Index (Lequesne et al. 1987). This Lequesne Index evaluates the symptoms of osteoarthritis concerning: (1) pain, such as nocturnal pain, or morning start pain etc., and (2) the mobility of the joints, such as the maximal walking distance after dosing of the pharmaceutical (Lequesne et al. 1987). With the help of the Lequesne Index, analgesic and/or anti-inflammatory effects of drugs can be recorded which are expressed as a relief from pain and an improvement in joint mobility. Nonsteroidal antiinflammatory drugs also improve these symptoms and perform well in such studies. Theoretically, morphine would also reduce the Lequesne Index because of its strong analgesic activity. Currently, a number of randomized, double-blind and placebo or nonsteroidal antiinflammatory drug controlled studies exist in which a reduction of the Lequesne Index or a similar complaint index was shown for all of the four medications discussed here; hence, improvements in mobility and relief of pain were shown by all these medications. All these clinical studies showed that these medications were well tolerated; amongst the reasons for this was the fact that the SYSADOAs do not inhibit cyclooxygenase. However, a certain risk arises from the use of hyaluronic acid since this agent has to be injected intra-articularly. As such, the risk for a joint infection has been estimated to be at between 1:10 000 and 1:30 000.

Finally, an analysis of pharmacological results from in vitro and animal experiments available until now has revealed that there is still a significant need for more preclinical investigations designed to show whether, and to what extent, these pharmaceuticals at clinically relevant concentrations act against the pathogenetically important processes occurring in osteoarthritic articular cartilage. They do, however, justify the statement that these agents are clinically effective concerning their abilities as "symptomatic slow acting drugs in osteoarthritis".

References

Akatsuka M, Yamamoto Y, Tobetto K, Yasui T, Ando T (1993) In vitro effects of hyaluronan on prostaglandin E2 induction by interleukin-1 in rabbit articular chondrocytes. Agents Action 38:122–125

Annefeld M, Fassbender HG (1983) Ultrastructural study of the activity of antiarthritic substances. Z Rheumatol 42:199–202

Armstrong S, Read R, Ghosh P (1994) The effects of intraarticular hyaluronan on cartilage and subchondral bone changes in an ovine model of early osteoarthritis. J Rheumatol 21:680–688

Bach G (1996) Arthrose-Medikamente mit verzögertem Wirkungseintritt. In: Gräfenstein K (ed) Therapie rheumatischer Erkrankungen. Ecomed, Landsberg/Lech, pp 66–70

Barcelo HA, Wiemeyer JC, Sagasta CL, Macias M, Barreira JC (1987) Effect of *S*-adenosylmethionine on experimental osteoarthritis in rabbits. Am J Med 83:55–59

Bassleer C, Reginster JY, Franchimont P (1993) Effects of glucosamine on differentiated human chondrocytes cultivated in clusters. Rev Esp Reumatol 20 [Suppl 1]:Mo 95

Dougados M (1996) On behalf of the Group for the Respect of Ethics and Excellence in Science (GREES), osteoarthritis section, Recommendations for the registration of drugs used in the treatment of osteoarthritis. Ann Rheum Dis 55:552–557

Engfeldt B, Hjertquist S-O (1967) The effect of various fixatives on the preservation of acid glycosaminoglycans in tissues. Pathol Microbiol Scand 171:219–232

Ghosh P, Holbert C, Read R, Armstrong S (1995) Hyaluronic acid (hyaluronan) in experimental osteoarthritis. J Rheumatol 43 [Suppl]:155–157

Ghosh P (1994) The role of hyaluronic acid (hyaluronan) in health and disease: interactions with cells, cartilage and components of synovial fluid. Clin Exp Rheum 12:75–82

Gotoh S, Miyazaki K, Onaya J, Sakamoto T, Tokuyasu K, Namiki O (1988) Experimental knee pain model in rats and analgesic effect of hyaluronate. Nippon Yakurigaku Zasshi 92:17–27

Gualano M, Berti F, Stramentinoli G (1985) Anti-inflammatory activity of *S*-adenosyl-L-methionine in animal models: possible interference with the eicosanoid system. Int J Tissue React 7:41–46

Harmand MF, Vilamitjana J, Maloche E, Duphil R, Ducassou D (1987) Effects of *S*-adenosylmethionine on human articular chondrocte differentiation. An in vitro study. Am J Med 83:48–54

Homandberg GA, Hui F, Wen C, Kuettner KE, Williams JM (1997) Hyaluronic acid suppresses fibronectin fragment mediated cartilage chondrolysis: I. In vitro. Osteoarthritis Cart 5:309–319

Hübner F, Steinmeyer J, Kalbhen DA (1997) Pharmacological influence on the collagenolytic activities of articular cartilage. Naunyn-Schmiedebergs Arch Pharmacol 355 [Suppl 4]:R87

Ialante A, Di Rosa M (1994) Hyaluronic acid modulates acute and chronic inflammation. Agents Actions 43:44–47

Ionac M, Parnham MJ, Plauchithiu M, Brune K (1996) Oxaceprol, an atypical inhibitor on inflammation and joint damage. Pharmacol Res 33:367–373

Jiménez SA, Dodge GR (1997) The effects of glucosamine sulfate (GS04) on human chondrocyte gene expression. Osteoarthritis Cart 5 [Suppl A]:72

Kalbhen DA, Jansen G (1990) Pharmacologic studies on the antidegenerative effect of ademetionine in experimental arthritis in animals. Arzneim-Forsch/Drug Res 40:1017–1021

Kalbhen DA, Kalkert B (1987) Autoradiography studies of the effect of oxaceprol on the metabolism of joint cartilage in vitro and in vivo. Z Rheumatol 46:136–142

Kalbhen DA (1987) Pharmakologische Untersuchungen mit chondroprotektiven Substanzen. In: Miehle W (ed) Chondroprotektion: Fakten und Aspekte. pmi Verlag, Frankfurt, pp 18–21

Kikuchi T, Yamada H, Shimmei M (1996) Effect of high molecular weight hyaluronan on cartilage degeneration in a rabbit model of osteoarthritis. Osteoarthritis Cart 4:99–110

Laurent UB, Fraser JR, Engstrom-Laurent A, Reed RK, Dahl LB, Laurent TC (1992) Catabolism of hyaluronan in the knee joint of the rabbit. Matrix 12:130–136

Lequesne M (1993) ILAR guidelines for testing slow acting drugs in osteoarthritis (SADOAs). Rev Esp Rumatol 20 [Suppl 1]:220–221
Lequesne MG, Mery C, Samson M, Gerard P (1987) Indexes of severity for osteoarthritis of the hip and knee. Scand J Rheumatol 65 [Suppl]:85–89
Mankin HJ, Brandt KD (1997) Pathogenesis of osteoarthritis. In: Kelley WN, Ruddy S, Harris ED, Sledge CB (eds) Textbook of rheumatology. WB Saunders, Philadelphia London, pp 1369–1382
Miyazaki K, Goto S, Okawara H (1984) Sodium hyaluronate (SPH): studies on analgesic and anti-inflammatory effects of sodium hyaluronate. Pharmacometrics 28:1123–1135
Morris EA, Wilcon S, Treadwell BV (1992) Inhibition of interleukin 1 mediated proteoglycan degradation in bovine articular cartilage explants by addition of sodium hyaluronate. Am J Vet Res 53:1977–1982
Nagase H, Okada Y (1997) Proteinases and matrix degradation. In: Kelley WN, Ruddy S, Harris ED, Sledge CB (eds) Textbook of rheumatology. WB Saunders, Philadelphia London, pp 323–342
Pelletier J-M, Martel-Pelletier J (1993) The pathophysiology of osteoarthritis and the implication of the use of hyaluronan and hylan as therapeutic agents in viscosupplementation. J Rheumatol 20:19–24
Pelletier JP, Howell DS (1993) Etiopathogenesis of osteoarthritis. In: McCarthy DJ, Koopman WJ (eds) Arthritis and allied conditions. Lea and Febiger, Philadelphia London, pp 1723–1734
Raiss R (1985) Effect of D-glucosamine sulfate on experimentally injured articular cartilage. Comparative morphometry of the ultrastructure of chondrocytes. Fortschr Med 103:658–662
Riera H, Aprile F, Mitrovic D (1990) Effect of oxaceprol on the proteoglycan and protein synthesis and degradation by cultured calf articular cartilage explants. Rev Rhum 57:579–583
Sandy JD, Flannery CR, Neame PJ, Lohmander LS (1992) The structure of aggrecan fragments in human synovial fluid. Evidence for the involvement in osteoarthritis of a novel proteinase which cleaves the Glu 373-Ala 374 bond of the interglobular domain. J Clin Invest 89:1512–1516
Setnikar I, Cereda R, Pacini MA, Revel L (1991) Antireactive properties of glucosamine sulfate. Arzneim-Forsch/Drug Res 41:157–161
Setnikar I, Pacini MA, Revel L (1991) Antiarthritic effects of glucosamine sulfate studied in animal models. Arzneim-Forsch/Drug Res 41:542–545
Shimazu A, Jikko A, Iwamoto M, Koike T, Yan W, Okada Y, Shinmei M, Nakamura S, Kato Y (1993) Effects of hyaluronic acid on the release of proteoglycan from the cell matrix in rabbit chondrocyte cultures in the presence and absence of cytokines. Arthritis Rheum 36:247–253
Shimizu C, Yoshioka M, Coutts RD, Harwood FL, Kubo T, Hirasawa Y, Amiel D (1998) Long-term effects of hyaluronan on experimental osteoarthritis in the rabbit knee. Osteoarthritis Cart 6:1–9
Steinmeyer J, Daufeldt S (1997) Pharmacological influence of antirheumatic drugs on the proteoglycans from interleukin-1 treated articular cartilage. Biochem Pharmacol 53:1627–1635
Steinmeyer J, Kim C, Sadowski T, Kalbhen DA (1996) Pharmacological influence on the activity of plasmin and plasminogen activators in vitro. Naunyn-Schmiedebergs Arch Pharmacol 353 [Suppl 4]:R7
Stramentinoli G (1987) Pharmacologic aspects of *S*-adenosylmethionine. Pharmacokinetics and pharmacodynamics. Am J Med 83:35–42
Tanaka S, Kumano F, Takayama M, Fukuda K (1997) Hyaluronic acid increases proteoglycan synthesis in articular cartilage degraded by interleukin-1. Osteoarthritis Cart 5 [Suppl A]:66

Vivien D, Galéra P, Loyau G, Pujol J-P (1993) *N*-acetyl-4-hydroxyproline (Oxaceprol®) and collagen synthesis in cultured synovial cells and articular cartilage. Osteoarthritis Cart 1:40

Weischer CH (1987) Antinozizeptive und antiinflammatorische Wirkung von *S*-Adenosylmethionin (SAMe) nach ein- und mehrmaliger intraperitonealer Applikation. In: Bach GL, Miehlke K (eds) Arthrose Workshop über Gumbaral® (Ademetionin). pmi-Verlag, Frankfurt, pp 81–86

Yasui T, Akatsuka M, Tobetto K, Umemoto J, Ando T, Yamashita K, Hayakawa T (1992) Effects of hyaluronan on the production of stromelysin and tissue inhibitor of metalloproteinase-1 (TIMP-1) in bovine articular chondrocytes. Biomed Res 13:343–348

Yoshioka M, Shimizu C, Harwood FL, Coutts RD, Amiel D (1997) The effect of hyaluronan during the development of osteoarthritis. Osteoarthritis Cart 5:257–260

Drug Treatment of Osteoarthritis: Clinical Aspects

K. K. Förster

Osteoarthritis (OA), degenerative joint disease, is a degenerative disease of the cartilage of the joints. The etiology is diverse and the pathogenesis unknown. The disease is clinically characterized by joint pain, tenderness, limitation of movement, occasional effusions, variable degrees of local inflammation, but without systemic manifestations, and therapeutically characterized by a lack of specific healing of articular cartilage damage (Mankin et al. 1986).

Taking this above cited definition of OA into account, it is understandable that patients with degenerative joint disease receive – for the most part – a variety of symptomatic treatments, including physiotherapy as well as medical and surgical measures. Therapy includes providing information to patients about their disease, and explanation of the available therapeutic alternatives. Concerning pharmacotherapy, today there are many drugs that are able to alleviate the symptoms of patients with OA, particularly in the knee or hip and in the initial stages, and thus provide the possibility to perform additional motion exercises and other physiotherapeutic measures. This will optimize joint function, and improve the patient's quality of life (Förster et al. 1997).

Historically, OA has been viewed as a natural sequel to aging or injury and as a disease for which little can be done to block its progression. Over the last two decades, however, the concept that pharmacological agents can be developed that at least conserve or even stimulate normal cartilage repair within the osteoarthritic joint has evolved (Howell et al. 1995). Up to now the significant increase in understanding of how growth factors and cytokines affect chondrocyte metabolism has substantially increased the number of potential targets for drug intervention in OA (Howell et al. 1995). However, specific therapy of osteoarthritis still lacks proof. Treatment with a demonstrable cause and effect relationship on the pathological process has still not been shown conclusively in the clinical arena.

The use of symptom relieving medicinal agents in the treatment of OA changed during the last decade, from completely empirical compounds such as cartilage extracts (e.g., Burkhardt and Ghosh 1987) to chemically defined substances. It has progressed from therapies with proof of effects primarily on the basis of preclinical tests and examinations to drugs with a thorough scientific background, based on confirmatory clinical studies.

In order to clearly define the objectives and to study the different claims for drugs used in osteoarthritis therapy, groups from different international scientific societies recently met. It was proposed that osteoarthritis drugs should be divided into two classes (Dougados et al. 1996): 1. Symptom modifying drugs; these act on symptoms with no detectable effect on the structural changes of the disease. 2. Structure modifying drugs; these interfere with the progression of the pathological changes observed in osteoarthritis. They can be further subclassified with respect to symptoms: (a) Structure modifying, symptom relieving drugs; (b) Structure modifying drugs with no independent effects on symptoms.

According to this classification, one would, for instance, assume that steroidal (corticosteroids) and nonsteroidal anti-inflammatory drugs (NSAIDs) primarily are symptom modifying drugs (class 1). On the other hand, it is under discussion that at least some of them may have an effect on hyaline cartilage – apart from the fact that this may be a negative effect (e.g. Rashad et al. 1989). These drugs should therefore belong to class 2a. To avoid such considerations and conflicts of classification respectively, it seems more appropriate to distinguish between symptom modifying and structure modifying effectiveness (activity) of a drug. This would at last mean that a substance or drug may show either symptom modifying or structure modifying activity, or even both activities (Förster et al. 1997) – as is the understanding also during the following expositions.

Symptom Modifying OA Drugs

Corticosteroids

Corticosteroids inhibit the activity of phospholipase A_2, which reduces the release of arachidonic acid. Thus, corticosteroids ultimately inhibit the formation of prostaglandins, thromboxane and the leukotrienes. Corticosteroids thus possess anti-inflammatory, anti-allergic and membrane-stabilizing properties.

Evidence exists to suggest that pro-inflammatory mediators are involved in cytokine-mediated cartilage resorption, implying that suppression by corticosteroids should be regarded as desirable (Morand 1997).

Corticosteroid therapy of osteoarthritis – by means of intra-articular injection of steroids – certainly provides temporary symptomatic relief. Trials have shown that the effect in the knee joint is only modest and very short-lived; the thumb base OA appears to respond better. All in all, it should be stressed that intra-articular steroids are of much less value in osteoarthritis than, for example, in rheumatoid arthritis (Bird 1991). The usual adverse systemic effects of corticosteroids during long-term use are not important after local therapy of OA. The risk of cartilage damage has been reviewed elsewhere (Wright 1978).

In common practice, intra-articular corticosteroids are probably justified in the following three situations in the management of OA, and the last indication is considered to be the most important (Dieppe 1994):

- Severe symptoms arising from the carpometacarpal joint of the thumb
- Flare-up of OA associated with a joint effusion
- As an adjunct to physical therapy.

Classical Nonsteroidal Anti-inflammatory Drugs

The use of classical nonsteroidal anti-inflammatory drugs (NSAIDs), depends on their analgesic (anti-nociceptive) and anti-inflammatory actions. They reduce pain, decrease gelling phenomenon, reduce occasional inflammation, and improve function in patients with osteoarthritis. The history of their therapeutic use spans more than 100 years. It was proposed that the mechanism of action is by inhibition of prostaglandin production through cyclooxygenase inhibition (Vane 1971).

The wide choice of classical NSAIDs requires classification. A common method is based upon the chemical structure. The therapeutic response is not closely linked to this but the adverse effects of the drug are rather more closely related to the chemical structure (Table 1).

Table 1. Classification of classical nonsteroidal anti-inflammatory drugs (NSAIDs) by structure (modified from Bird 1991)

Arylcarboxylic acids
Salicylic acids (acetylsalicylic acid, salsalate)
Anthranilic acid (mefenamic acid)
Arylalkanoic acids
Aryl propionic acids (ibuprofen, flurbiprofen, ketoprofen, naproxen, fenbufen, tiaprofenic acid)
Indole/indene acetic acids (indomethacin, proglumetacin, acemetacin, sulindac)
Heteroaryl acetic acid (tolmetin)
Phenyl acetic acid (diclofenac, aceclofenac)
Pyrano-carboxylic acid (etodolac)
Enolic acids
Pyrazolidinediones (phenylbutazone, oxyphenbutazone)
Benzotriazine (azapropazone)
Oxicame (piroxicam, tenoxicam, meloxicam)
Non-acidic agents
Naphthylalkanone (nabumetone)

Table 2. Classification of classical NSAIDs by half-life [modified from Mathies (1984)]

Short half-life (3–5 h)
Acetylsalicylic acid
Tiaprofenic acid
Ibuprofen
Indomethacin
Flufenamic acid
Aceclofenac
Diclofenac
Flurbiprofen
Acemetacin
Ketoprofen
Medium half-life group (5 to approximately 9 h)
Sulindac
Lonazolac
Pirprofen
Proglumetacin
Intermediate half-life (approximately 12 h)
Carprofen
Diflunisal
Azapropazone
Proquazone
Naproxen
Long half-life (20–45 h)
Kebuzon
Piroxicam
Meloxicam
Isoxicam
Very long half-life (60 h and more)
Oxyphenbutazone
Phenylbutazone
Oxaprozin
Tenoxicam

An alternative classification of NSAIDs is based on their half-life (Table 2) and may be of more practical value (Bird 1991).

In view of the discovery that there are at least two cyclooxygenase isoenzymes (COX-1, COX-2) and that preferential, and even selective, COX-2-inhibitors have been developed, the classification of NSAIDs according to their relative inhibition of cyclooxygenase isoenzymes (Frölich 1997) may provide an appropriate classification in the near future.

All classical NSAIDs have a common mechanism of action – inhibition of prostaglandin synthetase – though other mechanisms such as the inhibition of free oxygen radicals may also play a part. Some NSAIDs have been implicated in the possible inhibition of cytokine release though this would seem to be of greater benefit in purely inflammatory conditions such as rheumatoid arthritis rather than in osteoarthritis (Bird 1991). On the other hand, and based on preclinical investigations, other NSAIDs have been accused of causing deterioration in hyaline cartilage turnover. This is at least a cause for concern among strong inhibitors of prostaglandin synthetase – and may be of clinical importance (Rashad et al. 1989).

Balanced against the indisputable therapeutic value of NSAIDs – at least during short-term application – there is concern about adverse effects following the use of these drugs, especially in the elderly, in patients with known gastrointestinal problems, and in patients with impaired hepatic and renal function.

Simple Analgesics

Attempts to reduce these potential safety problems have led, among other considerations, to the question as to whether the anti-inflammatory effect of NSAIDs is necessary in every case of therapy. Painful OA, without a noticeable inflammatory component, could alternatively be treated with simple analgesics – such as paracetamol (acetaminophen), low dose salicylates or ibuprofen – without substantially inhibiting endogenous prostaglandin synthesis (Brune and Schmidt 1994). Recommendations to use analgesics as first choice in the treatment of OA is supported by traditional experience. In addition, the results of a clinical study of 4 weeks' duration confirm the clinical impression. Acetaminophen (4000 mg/day), a low (i.e. essentially analgesic) dose and a higher (i.e. anti-inflammatory) dose of ibuprofen induced equivalent changes of several OA indicators, including pain relief, in patients with OA of the knee (Bradley et al. 1991). On the other hand paracetamol often proves ineffective unless the OA is early and mild, and does have potential side effects (Bird 1991). So, this alternative way of drug treatment of OA patients remains controversial.

Nonclassical Nonsteroidal Anti-inflammatory Drugs

Besides corticosteroids, classical NSAIDs, and simple analgesics, current symptomatic pharmacotherapy of OA includes further substances and drugs with symptom relieving efficacy (Table 3).

Some of these drugs are examined in more detail below. They show – without exception – an anti-inflammatory effect that was shown in several models of inflammation, but unlike classical NSAIDs most of them do not inhibit cyclooxygenase or lipoxygenase. Therefore, they have been described as nonclassic NSAIDs (Di Pasquale 1993).

Table 3. Drugs used in the management of osteoarthritis (modified from Dieppe 1994)

Drug	Rationale/purpose
Simple analgesics	Pain relief
NSAIDs	Pain relief, reduction of other symptoms via anti-inflammatory effect
Intra-articular corticosteroids and other local applications	Local relief of symptoms
Intra-articular radiocolloids and sclerosing agents	Symptomatic relief via obliteration of the synovium and synovitis
Nonclassical NSAIDs	Symptom relief (and reduction in the progression of cartilage damage)
Antidepressants and other agents	Relief of pain

Ademetionin

Ademetionin (CAS-N°: 29908–03–0; MW 398.4) has the structural formula shown in Fig. 1. Ademetionin (*S*-Adenosyl-L-methionin; SAMe), a normal constituent of cells, is synthesized enzymatically from methionine and adenosine triphosphate (ATP) and is involved in various metabolic processes, probably including the sulfation of proteoglycans (Fife and Brandt 1992). As the tosilate-bis(sulphate)-salt (MW 766.9), the drug is available in Germany (Gumbaral) and Italy (Samyr) and is used in the therapy of depression, metabolic disorders, and musculoskeletal and joint disorders (Martindale 1993).

The pharmacologic characteristics seem to be relevant to its use in the treatment of osteoarthritis (Di Padova 1987). The results of animal experiments have shown that SAMe exerts anti-inflammatory and analgesic effects, but it does not seem to share with classical NSAIDs a common effect on the eicosanoid system, so that the mechanism of its pharmacologic action remains unclear. In addition, SAMe appears to enhance native proteoglycan synthesis and secretion in human chondrocyte cultures arising from the cartilage of patients with OA.

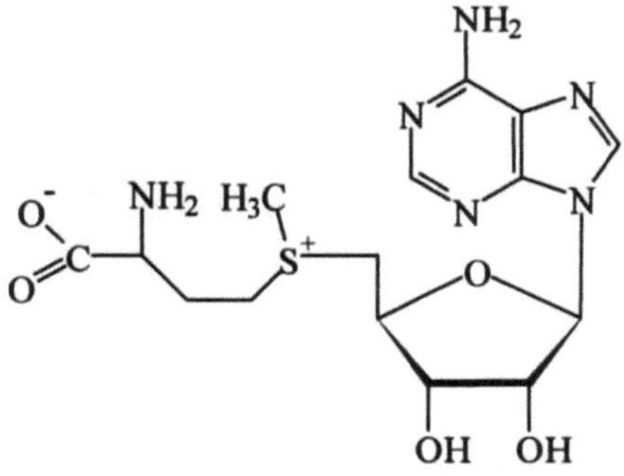

Fig. 1. Ademetionin

A number of clinical studies have been performed and more than 21 500 involved patients have been treated with SAMe, according to a review (Di Padova 1987). However, there is only one 3-week placebo controlled study in 76 patients concerning ademetionin's proof of efficacy in rheumatic disorders, especially in OA (Montrone et al. 1985). The authors themselves state that the results are only preliminary and that no definitive conclusions can be drawn. A further 4-week placebo and naproxen controlled study in 734 patients (Caruso and Pietrogrande 1987) also produced – from a statistical point of view – a result only of exploratory value. Today, more than 10 years later, there is still no clinical study that definitely confirms the symptom modifying activity of SAMe in patients with OA.

Chondroitin Sulfate

Chondroitin sulfate (ChS), is the sodium salt (CAS-N°: 9007–28–7; MW 50 000; sodium chondroitin sulfate) of a mixture of chondroitin-4-sulfate and chondroitin-6-sulfate. The latter has the structural formula shown in Fig. 2. ChS, a constituent of the cartilaginous matrix, is available in many parts of the world, for instance in Austria (Condrosulf), France (e.g. Chondrosulf), Italy, Spain, and Switzerland (Condrosulf, Structum), USA and Canada. It is used in the therapy of degenerative joint disorders.

Its structural and pharmacokinetic characterization has been reported (Conte et al. 1995). ChS was said to cause an increase in RNA synthesis by the chondrocytes, which appears to correlate with an increase in the synthesis of proteoglycans and collagens (Morreale et al. 1996). In addition, there is evidence to indicate that ChS partially inhibits leukocyte elastase activity (Baici and Bradamante 1984) and that it possesses anti-inflammatory activity (Ronca et al. 1998).

Concerning the proof of the clinical efficacy of ChS there are results of placebo-controlled studies (e.g. L'Hirondel 1992; Mazières et al. 1992), but German health authorities, for instance, did not accept them as definitive. Registration in Germany has been refused (BfArM 1994).

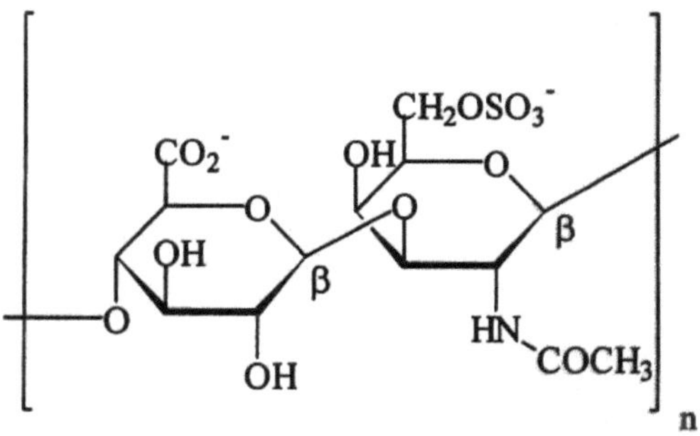

Fig. 2. Chondroitin sulfate

Since then several other clinical studies have been performed. The first study with a duration of 6 months compared the clinical efficacy of ChS (3 months treatment) to diclofenac sodium and placebo in 146 patients with knee OA. It showed an interesting, continuous therapeutic effect of ChS over 3 months after discontinuation of treatment (Morreale et al. 1996).

There are a further four recently published placebo-controlled studies. Two of these studies, with a duration of 3 months (Bourgeois et al. 1998) and 6 months (Bucsi and Poór 1998), respectively, showed a symptomatic efficacy of ChS in 207 (completed) patients with OA of the knee. However, statistically they are only of exploratory value. The other two studies – one study in 119 patients with finger joint OA, who were followed for 3 years (Verbruggen et al. 1998), and the other in 42 patients with knee OA, who were treated and followed for 1 year (Uebelhart et al. 1998) – were described as pilot studies (i.e. they also are only of preliminary character). Nevertheless, it was discussed that ChS might be capable of influencing the natural course of the degenerative disease (Uebelhart et al. 1998).

Diacerein

Diacerein (CAS-N°: 13739-02-1; MW 368.3) is a low molecular weight heterocyclic compound (anthroic acid derivative) with the structural formula shown in Fig. 3. Diacerein (Diacerhein, Diacetylrhein) is used as diacetate salt in the management of OA and is available in France (ART 50) and Switzerland (e.g. Artrodar), for example.

Following absorption diacerein is rapidly broken down into its active metabolite, rhein. Pharmacodynamically, diacerein shows anti-inflammatory and analgesic properties, stimulates collagen and glycosaminoglycan synthesis by chondrocytes, inhibits interleukin-1 induced collagenolysis, superoxide production, and lipid peroxidation, without affecting endogenous prostaglandin or leukotriene synthesis (Trans Bussan 1996).

There are three placebo controlled clinical studies (according to Trans Bussan 1996), but only one of them has been published recently (Nguyen et al. 1994). A total of 288 patients with OA of the hip were treated for

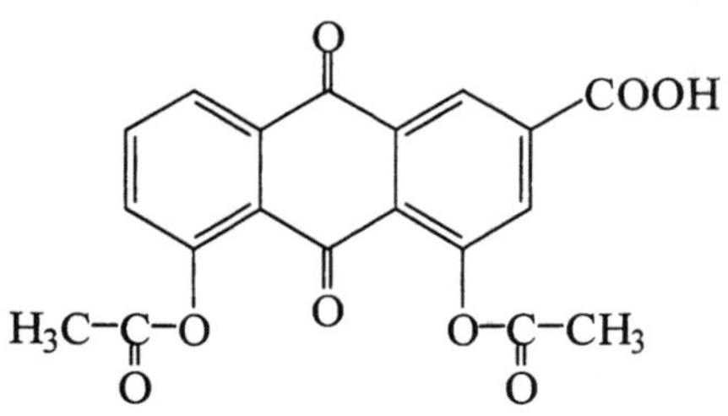

Fig. 3. Diacerein

2 months either with diacerein, tenoxicam, a combination of both, or with placebo. Even though the active treatments appeared to be superior to placebo in the improvement of symptoms (pain score, joint function), the study is – from a statistical point of view – a pilot study and the results are therefore only preliminary.

Glucosamine Sulfate

Glucosamine sulfate (CAS-N°: 14999–43–0; MW 456.4), the sulphuric acid salt of the amino-monosaccharide glucosamine (CAS-N°: 3416–24–8; MW 179.2), is a chemically small and well-characterized molecule, which has the structural formula shown in Fig. 4.

Glucosamine, which is found physiologically in the connective tissues of the human body, represents the preferred substrate in the biosynthesis of glycosaminoglycans (hyaluronic acid, chondroitin sulfate, keratane sulfate) of the hyaline cartilage and the synovia. The sulfate (GS) is available as drug in Germany (Dona 200-S), Italy (Dona), Spain (Xicil), Portugal (Viartril) as well as in other countries (in USA, Canada, Asia, Eastern Europe and South America) and is used in the treatment of OA.

Based on its pharmacokinetic pattern, pharmacodynamically GS increases anabolic mechanisms, as shown, for instance, in vitro by proteoglycan synthesis stimulation in chondrocytes isolated from human OA articular cartilage (Bassleer et al. 1998), increases chondrocyte adhesion to fibronectin (Piperno et al. 1998), reduces catabolic mechanisms and exerts cyclooxygenase independent anti-inflammatory actions in different experimental inflammatory models (Setnikar et al. 1991 a; Setnikar et al. 1991 b).

Approximately 30 clinical trials involving about 8000 OA patients document the ability of GS to diminish the symptoms of the disease (pain and movement limitation). Symptom modifying activity was definitely proven in short-term, placebo-controlled randomized, double-blind clinical studies involving 407 patients with osteoarthritis of the knee (Noack et al. 1994; Reichelt et al. 1994). A further well-designed and performed study of 5 months duration in 329 patients with OA of the knee (Bourgeois et

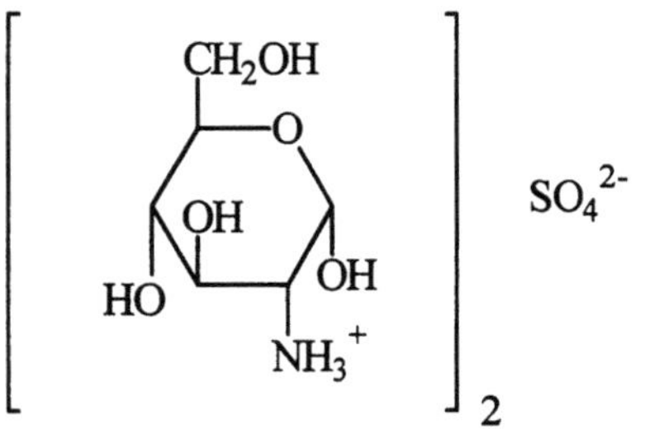

Fig. 4. Glucosamine sulfate

al. 1999) confirmed the results that GS is significantly more effective than placebo in the control of OA symptoms and as safe as placebo. Compared to NSAIDs, GS is equally effective and significantly safer (Bourgeois et al. 1999). Studies in OA of other joints have already been published (Giacovelli and Rovati 1993) or are still in progress. Because of its long-lasting symptom relieving efficacy after discontinuation of therapy, GS has been or is currently being studied in trials of long-term duration (1–3 years) to confirm its clinical activity over this time and to test its potential as a symptom modifying OA drug with additional structure modifying activity.

Hyaluronic Acid

Hyaluronic acid (CAS-N°: 9004-61-9; molecular weight 50 000–8 000 000), applied as sodium salt (CAS-N°: 9067-32-7; hyaluronate sodium), has the structural formula shown in Fig. 5.

The macromolecule hyaluronic acid (HA) is present in the hyaline cartilage linked to proteoglycans. It is the viscosity determining factor in the joint fluid. HA has always been assumed to function as a lubricant. The idea of "viscosupplementation" (Balazs and Denlinger 1993) has successfully led to the introduction of HA as a drug (Hyalart, Hyalgan) and as a medical device (Synvisc) for intra-articular application. HA is on the market, for example, in North America, Austria, Germany, Switzerland and other countries.

Concerning pharmacology, in vitro studies have shown that HA possesses an anti-inflammatory effect including inhibition of chemotaxis of inflammatory cells, removal of free oxygen radicals and inhibition of prostaglandin synthesis. The pharmacologic and visco-rheologic basis (Balazs and Denlinger 1993) as well as the wealth of therapeutic experience have been extensively reviewed (Peyron 1993; Maheu 1995).

Symptom modifying activity was confirmed, for example, in one prospective multicenter, double-blind study (Puhl et al. 1993) in 209 patients

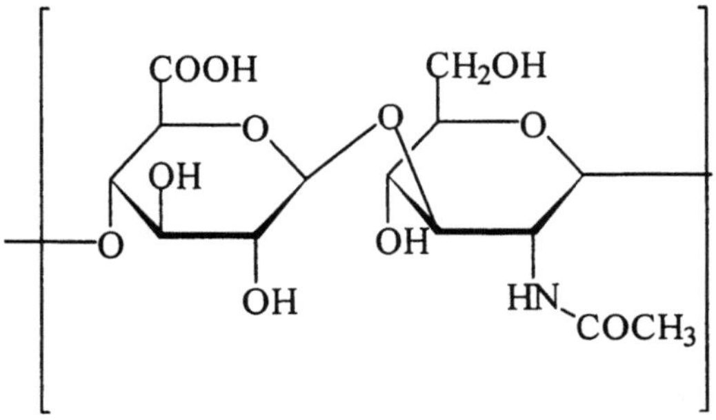

Fig. 5. Hyaluronic acid

with OA of the knee, who were treated for 5 weeks (one injection per week) with either 25 mg or HA placebo (0.25 mg HA). The algofunctional Lequesne Index (Lequesne et al. 1987), the main evaluation parameter, showed a statistically significant superiority of the treated patients after the third injection up to the final examination, 9 weeks after the last injection (Puhl et al. 1993). On the other hand, another study of 20 weeks observation duration assessed the effect of HA on knee OA symptoms in 240 patients and could not show a difference between unstratified groups treated with either placebo or HA. However, comparison of treatment groups stratified by age and baseline algofunctional index revealed a significant difference in favor of HA over placebo (pain, activity, algofunctional index, global evaluations by patient and investigator) for patients older than 60 years and a baseline index greater than 10 (Lohmander et al. 1996).

There are a few pilot studies evaluating HA's potential structure modifying activity, e.g. a 1-year arthroscopically controlled study in 39 patients (Listrat et al. 1997) and an open microarthroscopic evaluation in 40 patients, 6 months after a series of five injections of HA (Frizziero et al. 1998), but definite conclusions cannot yet be drawn.

Oxaceprol

Oxaceprol (CAS-N°: 33996-33-7; MW 173.2) is the acetylated form of hydroxyproline, a non-essential amino acid, which is part of the collagen structures. Oxaceprol has the structural formula shown in Fig. 6. Oxaceprol (acetyl-hydroxy-L-proline) is available in France (Jonctum) and Germany (AHP 200) and is used in the treatment of inflammatory and degenerative joint diseases.

On the basis of preclinical examinations, Oxaceprol is said to stimulate the biosynthesis of collagen and glycosaminoglycans of hyaline cartilage and to possess an analgesic as well as a prostaglandin-independent anti-inflammatory effect (Menge 1995). In addition, oxaceprol is able to inhibit leukocyte infiltration and late connective tissue changes in experimental models of inflammatory joint disease (Ionac et al. 1996).

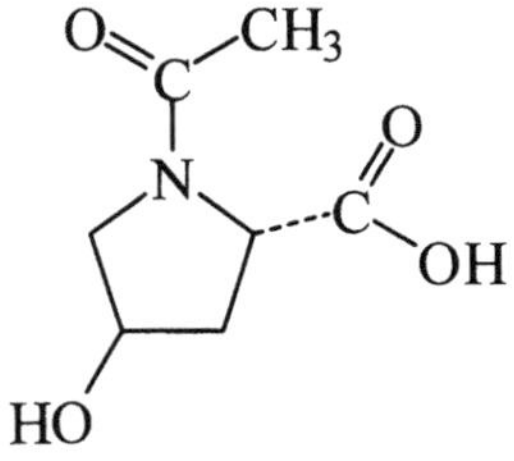

Fig. 6. Oxaceprol

Ten controlled clinical studies have been performed, seven studies (involving 685 patients) compared to the NSAIDs ibuprofen and diclofenac and three studies compared to placebo, respectively (Menge 1995). From the statistical point of view, all NSAID-controlled studies are performed inadequately. Their corresponding results, no statistically significant difference, therefore does not mean an equivalence between oxaceprol and ibuprofen or diclofenac. Concerning the placebo-controlled studies, two (involving 78 patients) show a superiority of oxaceprol, but design and implementation are not good enough for today's requirements (Menge 1995). A third study (6 months; prospective, randomized, double-blind), in 323 patients with OA of the knee or hip, could not show any difference between placebo, 600 mg/day oxaceprol, and 1200 mg/day oxaceprol in the main efficacy parameter (Dreiser et al. 1995). In conclusion, oxaceprol's symptom modifying activity has not yet been established in OA patients.

Structure (Disease) Modifying OA Drugs

Experience based on in vitro studies and animal models shows that some drugs used in the treatment of OA, rather than having a beneficial symptomatic effect, may accelerate or exacerbate the pathological changes of osteoarthritis (Brandt et al. 1998). That this may be also of clinical importance has been mentioned above regarding corticosteroids (Wright 1978) and NSAIDs (Rashad et al. 1989).

This potential drug induced cartilage change for the worse has stimulated interest in pharmacologic agents that may be able to positively influence the pathogenetic mechanisms in OA. If they reverse or at least retard the OA process, these agents would be disease modifying (Lequesne et al. 1994) or structure modifying drugs (Dougados et al. 1996).

There are a wealth of substances that have already been tested preclinically for structure modifying activity in osteoarthritis models (Table 4), concerning clinical proof however, so far a specific treatment of OA has not been confirmed in hypothesis testing studies.

But there are already a few published exploratory (pilot) clinical studies, testing drugs as to their structure modifying activity in OA. To date, chondroitin sulfate (Uebelhart et al. 1998), glucosamine sulfate (Reginster et al. 1999) and hyaluronic acid (Listrat et al. 1997) seem to be the most promising ones. Therefore, a future challenge in the area of OA research will be the design and implementation of appropriate and confirmatory clinical trials (Dieppe 1994) to prove whether or not they have a demonstrable causal effect on the pathological process judged by existing guidelines (Lequesne et al. 1994) and recommendations, respectively (Altman et al. 1996).

Table 4. Substances tested preclinically for disease-modifying activity in osteoarthritis models (modified from Altman and Howell 1998)

Sulfated glycosaminoglycans
Glycosaminoglycan peptide (GAG peptide)
Glycosaminoglycan polysulfuric acid (GAGPS)
Chondroitin sulfate (ChS)
Glucosamine sulfate (GS)
Non-sulfated glycosaminoglycans
Hyaluronic acid (HA)
Agents acting on bone
Bisphosphonates (Etidronate)
Calcitonin
Anti-inflammatory agents
NSAIDs
Glucocorticoids
Lipids
Enzyme inhibitors
Tetracyclines (Doxycycline)
Specific stromelysin inhibitors
Specific collagenase inhibitors
Cytokines, antagonists, growth factors
Growth hormone
Insulin-like growth factor-1 (IGF-1)
Transforming growth factor-beta (TGF-β)
Interleukin-1 receptor antagonist (IL-1ra)
Others
Diacerein (Diacerhein, Diacetylrhein)
Estrogens, Tamoxifen
Oxaceprol
S-adenosyl-L-methionine (SAMe)
Phytotherapeutics
Homeotherapy

References

Altman R, Brandt K, Hochberg M, Moskowitz R, et al. (1996) Design and conduct of clinical trials in patients with osteoarthritis: Recommendations from a task force of the Osteoarthritis Research Society. Osteoarthritis Cart 4:217–243

Altman RD, Howell DS (1998) Disease-modifying osteoarthritis drugs. In: Brandt KD, Doherty M, Lohmander LS (eds) Osteoarthritis. Oxford University Press, Oxford New York Toronto, pp 417–428

Baici A, Bradamante P (1984) Interaction between human leukocyte elastase and chondroitin sulfate. Chem Biol Interact 51:1–11

Balazs EA, Denlinger JL (1993) Viscosupplementation: a new concept in the treatment of osteoarthritis. J Rheumatol 20 [Suppl 39]:3–9

Bassleer C, Rovati L, Franchimont P (1998) Stimulation of proteoglycan production by glucosamine sulfate in chondrocytes isolated from human osteoarthritic articular cartilage in vitro. Osteoarthritis Cart 6:427–434

BfArM – German Federal Institute for Drugs and Medicinal Products (1994) Bekanntmachung über die Zulassung und Registrierung von Arzneimitteln (Aufbereitungsmonographien für den humanmedizinischen Bereich) Negativ-Monographie: Chondroitin sulfate mixture. Bundesanzeiger 46:10354

Bird H (1991) The current treatment of osteoarthritis. In: Russel RG, Dieppe P (eds) Osteoarthritis: current research and prospects for pharmacological intervention. IBC, London, pp 173–195

Bourgeois P, Chales G, Dehais J, Delcambre B, Kuntz J-L, Rozenberg S (1998) Efficacy and tolerability of chondroitin sulfate 1200 mg/day vs chondroitin sulfate 3×400 mg/day vs placebo. Osteoarthritis Cart 6 [Suppl A]:25–30

Bourgeois P, Giacovelli G, Rovati LC, Menkes C-J (1999) Effects of glucosamine sulfate on symptoms of knee osteoarthritis. N Engl J Med 341 (in press)

Bradley JD, Brandt KD, Katz BP, Kalasinski LA, Ryan SI (1991) Comparison of an antiinflammatory dose of ibuprofen, an analgesic dose of ibuprofen, and acetaminophen in the treatment of patients with osteoarthritis of the knee. N Engl J Med 325:87–91

Brandt K, Lohmander LS, Doherty M (1998) Prospects for pharmacological modification of joint breakdown in osteoarthritis. In: Brandt KD, Doherty M, Lohmander LS (eds) Osteoarthritis. Oxford University Press, Oxford New York Toronto, pp 415–417

Brune K, Schmidt N (1994) Nichtsteroidale Antiphlogistika. Neue Einsichten zu Wirkort und Wirkmechanismus. DAZ 134:3815–3817

Bucsi L, Poór G (1998) Efficacy and tolerability of oral chondroitin sulfate as a symptomatic slow-acting drug for osteoarthritis (SYSADOA) in the treatment of knee osteoarthritis. Osteoarthritis Cart 6 [Suppl A]:31–36

Burkhardt D, Ghosh P (1987) Laboratory evaluation of antiarthritic drugs as potential chondroprotective agents. Semin Arthritis Rheum 17 [Suppl 1]:3–34

Caruso I, Pietrogrande V (1987) Italian double-blind multicenter study comparing *S*-adenosylmethionine, naproxen, and placebo in the treatment of degenerative joint disease. Am J Med 83 [Suppl 5A]:66–71

Conte A, Volpi N, Palmieri L, Bahous I, Ronca G (1995) Biochemical and pharmacokinetic aspects of oral treatment with chondroitin sulfate. Arzneim-Forsch/Drug Res 45II:918–925

Dieppe P (1994) Osteoarthritis management. In: Klippel JH, Dieppe P (eds) Rheumatology. Mosby, St. Louis Baltimore Boston Chicago London Philadelphia Sydney Toronto, 7.8.1–7.8.8

Di Padova C (1987) *S*-Adenosylmethionine in the treatment of osteoarthritis. Am J Med 83 [Suppl 5A]:60–65

Di Pasquale G (1993) Pharmacological control of cartilage degradation in osteoarthritis. In: Woessner JF Jr, Howell DS (eds) Joint cartilage degradation. Marcel Dekker, New York Basel Hong Kong, pp 475–501

Dougados M, Devogelaer JP, Annefeld M, et al. on behalf of the Group for the Respect of Ethics and Excellence in Science (GREES), osteoarthritis section (1996) Recommendations for the registration of drugs used in the treatment of osteoarthritis. Ann Rheum Dis 55:552–557

Dreiser RL, Bonnet C, Marty M, Mazières B, Neveur C, Sebert JL, Vignon E (1995) A placebo-controlled double-blind study of Oxaceprol in the long-term treatment of osteoarthritis of the knee or the hip. Rheumatology in Europe 24 [Suppl 3]:331

Fife R, Brandt KD (1992) Other approaches to therapy. In: Moskowitz RW, Howell DS, Goldberg VM, Mankin HJ (eds) Osteoarthritis – diagnosis and medical/surgical management, 2nd edn. Saunders, Philadelphia London Toronto Montreal Sydney Tokyo, pp 511–526

Förster KK, Schmid K, Bach GL (1997) Current aspects of pharmacotherapy in osteoarthritis. arthritis + rheuma 17:23–28

Frizziero L, Govoni E, Bacchini P (1998) Intra-articular hyaluronic acid in the treatment of osteoarthritis of the knee: clinical and morphological study. Clin Exp Rheumatol 16:441–449

Frölich JC (1997) A classification of NSAIDs according to the relative inhibition of cyclooxygenase isoenzymes. Trends Pharmacol Sci 18:30–34

Giacovelli G, Rovati LC (1993) Clinical efficacy of glucosamine sulfate in osteoarthritis of the spine. Rev Esp Reumatol 20 [Suppl 1]:325

Howell DS, Altman RD, Pelletier J-P, Martel-Pelletier J, Dean DD (1995) Disease-modifying antirheumatic drugs: current status of their application in animal models of osteoarthritis. In: Kuettner KE, Goldberg VM (eds) (Supported by the American Academy of Orthopaedic Surgeons) Osteoarthritic Disorders. AAOS, Rosemont, IL, pp 365–377

Ionac M, Parnham MJ, Plauchithiu M, Brune K (1996) Oxaceprol, an atypical inhibitor of inflammation and joint damage. Pharmacol Res 33:367–373

Lequesne M, Mery C, Samson M, Gerard P (1987) Indexes of severity for osteoarthritis of the hip and knee: validation-value in comparison with other assessment tests. Scand J Rheumatol 16 [Suppl 65]:85–89

Lequesne M, Brandt KD, Bellamy N, Moskowitz R, Menkes CJ, Pelletier J-P et al. (1994) Guidelines for testing slow-acting and disease-modifying drugs in osteoarthritis. J Rheumatol 21 [Suppl 41]:65–71

L'Hirondel JL (1992) Klinische Doppelblind-Studie mit oral verabreichtem Chondroitinsulfat gegen Placebo bei der tibiofemoralen Gonarthrose (125 Patienten). In: Lequesne M, Lualdi P, Numo R (eds) Orales Chondroitinsulfat bei Arthrose. EULAR Verlag, Basel, pp 77–84

Listrat V, Ayral X, Patarnello F, Bonvarlet J-P, Simmonet J, Amor B, Dougados M (1997) Arthroscopic evaluation of potential structure modifying activity of hyaluronan (Hyalgan) in osteoarthritis of the knee. Osteoarthritis Cart 5:153–160

Lohmander LS, Dalen N, Englund G, et al. (1996) Intra-articular hyaluronan injections in the treatment of osteoarthritis of the knee: a randomised, double blind, placebo controlled multicentre trial. Hyaluronan Multicentre Trial Group. Ann Rheum Dis 55:424–431

Maheu E (1995) Hyaluronan in knee osteoarthritis: a review of the clinical trials with Hyalgan. Eur J Rheumatol Inflamm 15:17–24

Mankin HJ, Brandt KD, Shulman LE (1986) Workshop on etiopathogenesis of osteoarthritis. Proceedings and recommendations. J Rheumatol 13:1127–1160

Martindale W (1993) The extra pharmacopoeia, 30th Rev edn. Reynolds JEF (ed) Pharmaceutical Press, London, pp 1812

Mathies H (1984) Nichtsteroidale Antirheumatika. In: Mathies H (ed) Leitfaden für Diagnose und Therapie rheumatischer Erkrankungen. EULAR Verlag, Basel, pp 216–220

Mazières B, Loyau G, Menkès, Valat JP, Dreiser RL, Charlot J, Masounabe-Puyanne A (1992) Le chondroitine sulfate dans le traitment de la gonarthrose et de la coxarthrose. Rev Rhum Mal Ostéoartic 59:466–472

Menge M (1995) Oxaceprol im Spiegel der wissenschaftlichen Literatur (Oxaceprol in the mirror of the scientific literature; Clinical expert report). In: Chephasaar (ed) Med Info 1/95. St. Ingbert, Germany, pp 1–30

Montrone F, Fumagalli M, Sarzi-Puttini T, Boccassini L, Santandrea S, Volpato R, Locati M, Caruso I (1985) Double-blind study of *S*-adenosylmethionine versus placebo in hip and knee arthrosis. Clin Rheumatol 4:484–485

Morand E (1997) Corticosteroids in the treatment of rheumatologic diseases. Curr Opin Rheumatol 9:200–205

Morreale P, Manopulo R, Galati M, Boccanera L, Saponati G, Bocchi L (1996) Comparison of the anti-inflammatory osteoarthritis efficacy of chondroitin sulfate and diclofenac sodium in patients with knee. J Rheumatol 23:1385–1391
Nguyen M, Dougados M, Berdah L, Amor B (1994) Diacerhein in the treatment of osteoarthritis of the hip. Arthritis Rheum 37:529–536
Noack W, Fischer M, Förster KK, Rovati LC, Setnikar I (1994) Glucosamine sulfate in osteoarthritis of the knee. Osteoarthritis Cart 2:51–59
Peyron JG (1993) A new approach to the treatment of osteoarthritis: viscosupplementation. Osteoarthritis Cart 1:85–87
Piperno M, Reboul P, Hellio le Graverand M-P, Peschard MJ, Annefeld M, Richard M, Vignon E (1998) Osteoarthritic cartilage fibrillation is associated with a decrease in chondrocyte adhesion to fibronectin. Osteoarthritis Cart 6:393–399
Puhl W, Bernau A, Greiling H, Köpcke W, Pförringer W, Steck KJ, Zacher J, Scharf HP (1993) Intra-articular sodium hyaluronate in osteoarthritis of the knee: a multicenter, double-blind study. Osteoarthritis Cart 1:233–241
Rashad S, Revell P, Hemingway A, Low F, Rainsford K, Walker F (1989) Effect of non-steroidal anti-inflammatory drugs on the course of osteoarthritis. Lancet ii:519–522
Reginster JY, Deroisy R, Paul I, Lee RL, Henrotin Y, Giacovelli G, Dacre J, Rovati LC, Gosset C (1999) Glucosamine sulfate significantly reduces progression of knee osteoarthritis over 3 years: A large, randomised, placebo-controlled, double-blind, prospective trial (abstract). Oral presentation on the occasion of the 63rd ACR Meeting, Boston
Reichelt A, Förster KK, Fischer M, Rovati LC, Setnikar I (1994) Efficacy and safety of intramuscular glucosamine sulfate in osteoarthritis of the knee. Arzneim-Forsch/Drug Res 44I:75–80
Ronca F, Palmieri L, Panicucci P, Ronca G (1998) Anti-inflammatory activity of chondroitin sulfate. Osteoarthritis Cart 6 [Suppl A]:14–21
Setnikar I, Cereda R, Pacini MA, Revel L (1991) Antireactive properties of glucosamine sulfate. Arzneim-Forsch/Drug Res 41I:157–161
Setnikar I, Pacini MA, Revel L (1991) Antiarthritic effects of glucosamine sulfate studied in animal models. Arzneim-Forsch/Drug Res 41I:542–545
Trans Bussan (1996) Artrodar – Diacerein – new light in osteoarthritis. Product information brochure. Trans Bussan, Geneva, pp 3–26
Uebelhart D, Thonar EJ-MA, Delmas PD, Chantraine A, Vignon E (1998) Effects of oral chondroitin sulfate on the progression of knee osteoarthritis: a pilot study. Osteoarthritis Cart 6 [Suppl A]:39–46
Vane J (1971) Inhibition of prostaglandin synthesis as mechanism of action for aspirin-like drugs. Nature New Biol 231:232–235
Verbruggen G, Goemaere S, Veys EM (1998) Chondroitin sulfate: S/DMOAD (structure/disease modifying anti-osteoarthritis drug) in the treatment of finger joint AO. Osteoarthritis Cart 6 [Suppl A]:37–38
Wright V (1978) Intra-articular steroids. BMJ 1:600–601

Histological Changes of Cartilage and Subchondral Bone in Varus Gonarthrosis: Comparison with Radiographic and Macroscopic Findings

H. Reichel and M. Hein

Introduction

The initial pathomorphological changes in osteoarthrosis can be located in the joint cartilage (calcified and noncalcified hyaline cartilage), in the subchondral bone, or in the synovial membrane (Fig. 1). Depending on the particular reason, primarily mechanical-induced or an enzyme-induced cartilage damage is produced (Hackenbroch 1992). The reason for the mechanically induced cartilage damage is a pathological load distribution in the knee joint, which leads to local cartilage overload and exceeds the tolerance threshold of the joint cartilage. A varus deviation of the mechanical axis results in a greater overload in the medial compartment of the knee joint, followed by a varus gonarthrosis. It is presumed that the enzyme-induced cartilage destruction, produces an intraarticular release of enzymes and inflammation mediators, which in turn decrease the cartilage resistance below the level necessary for everyday joint loading.

Both the mechanical and the enzyme-induced cartilage damage disturb the balance between loading and loading capacity. For the ensuing pathogenetic process of osteoarthrosis, the strain put on the already damaged joint at a particular time is important. Beside the joint loading, other mod-

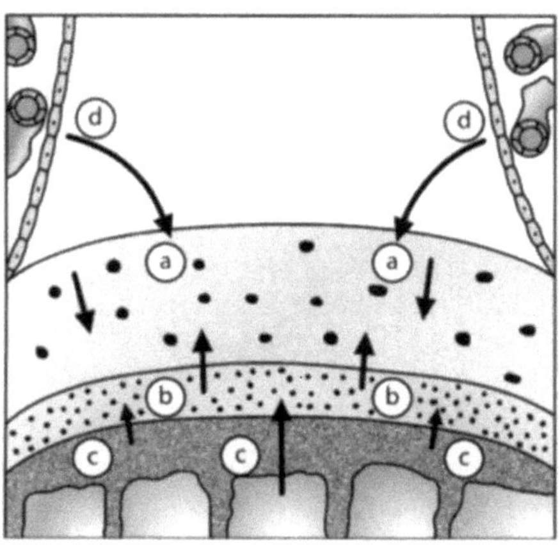

Fig. 1. Initial localizations of knee osteoarthrosis. Noncalcified hyaline cartilage (*a*), calcified hyaline cartilage (*b*), subchondral bone (*c*), or synovial membrane (*d*)

ifying factors of osteoarthrosis are: immobility, individual stress intolerance, pregnancy, environmental and climate factors (Hackenbroch 1992).

Early Stages of Knee Osteoarthrosis

Early signs can be seen in the superficial layers of the hyaline cartilage. Because of the disturbance of chondrocyte synthesis or degradative enzymes of the synovial fluid, a superficial loss of proteoglycans can be observed (Fig. 2). At the same time, breakage and loosening of the collagen

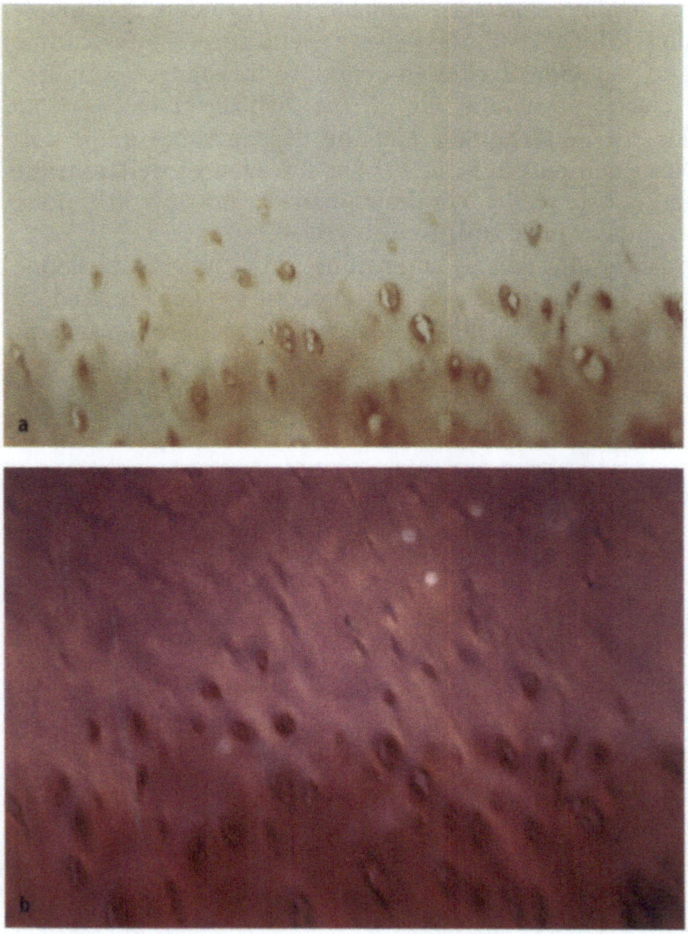

Fig. 2 a, b. Lateral tibial base plate in moderate varus gonarthrosis. Safranin-O staining, ×100. Distinct loss of proteoglycans, in light microscopy. **a** No structures in superficial layers. **b** The polarization microscopy shows the superficial layers poor in proteoglycans

fibers starts to appear in the tangential cartilage layers (Sokoloff 1980). These fibrillations are the macroscopic correlation of errors and changes in the fibrous network, caused either mechanically or by incorrect production of collagen types I and III (von der Mark 1986). The breakage of the collagen network leads to larger pores and allows an increased inflow of water and other molecules into the cartilage. After the fibrillation of the cartilage surface, fissures and cracks occur vertically and obliquely on the surface, some of them even reaching the tidemark. The consequence is a significant change in the biomechanical properties of the cartilage. The response to the changed loading conditions is a distinct widening of the ossified cartilage layer. The tidemark, the border line between calcified and noncalcified cartilage, can show duplication (Fig. 3).

In principle, the hyaline cartilage is unable to regenerate; healing of defects is impossible (Stiller 1982). However, reparative processes can be observed parallel to the loss of chondrocytes. By division of chondrocytes and by cell cluster formation (Fig. 4), the cartilage tissue starts to compensate the loss of proteoglycans and the degeneration of the collagen network (Dustmann and Puhl 1978). But the change-over from the reversible postmitotic state to the synthesis phase is too slow; therefore, it is a quantitatively inadequate substitution.

To increase formation of cartilage, an opening of the subchondral bone marrow is necessary. The cartilage defect region can then be replaced by fibrous tissue, which is subsequently transformed into fibrous cartilage (Fig. 5). However, the mechanical properties of this cartilage replacement are inadequate for longer survival; the fibrous cartilage becomes a victim

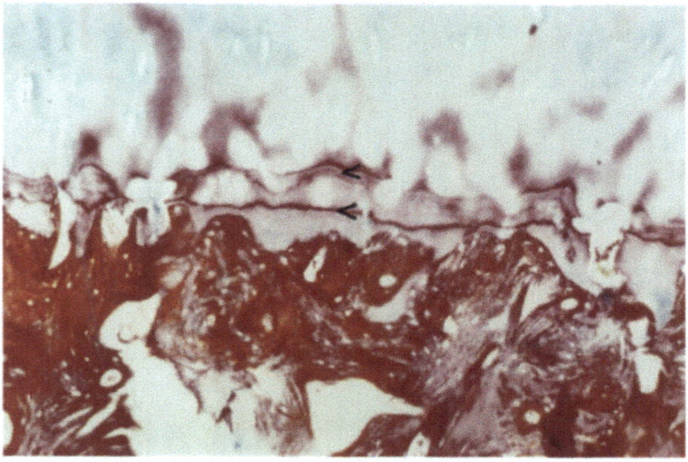

Fig. 3. Medial tibial base plate in moderate varus gonarthrosis. Azan staining, ×100. The reduced energy-absorptive capacity of the degenerated cartilage leads to widening of the calcified cartilage zone with duplication of the tidemark (*arrows*) and hyperostosis of the subchondral bone

of abrasion and degeneration (Otte 1974). This substitution is qualitatively inadequate. In cases of enzymatic cartilage degeneration, the reduced reparative capacity of the tissue results in a rapid cartilage loss without morphological adaptations.

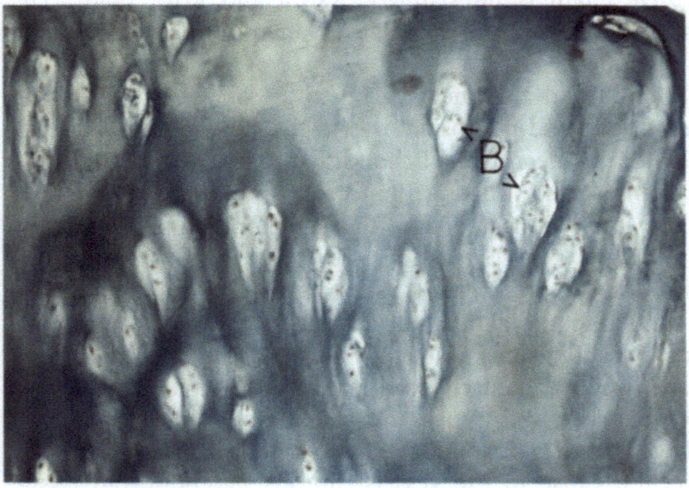

Fig. 4. Medial femoral condyle in moderate varus gonarthrosis. Azan staining, ×100. Cell clusters (*B*) of ten and more chondrocytes in unmasked hyaline cartilage, poor in stained base substance

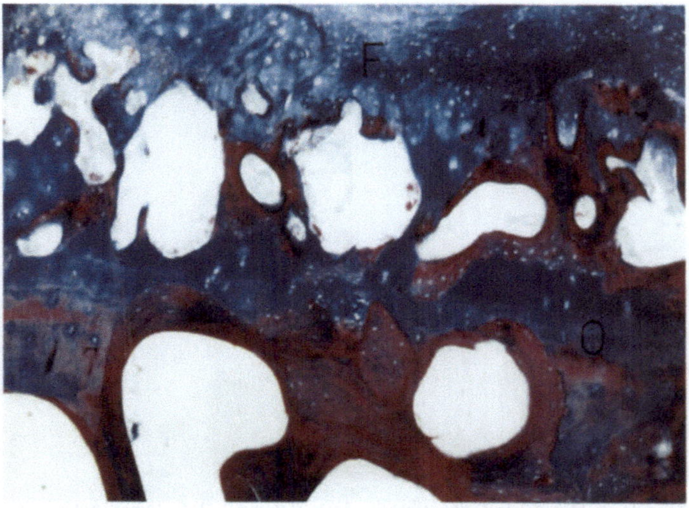

Fig. 5. Medial tibial base plate in moderate varus gonarthrosis. Azan staining, ×75. Regenerates of fibrous cartilage (*F*) above the original calcified hyaline cartilage (*O*)

Late Stages of Knee Osteoarthrosis

In later stages progressive cartilage abrasion leads to successive loss of noncalcified and calcified cartilage (Fig. 6). Caused by increased loading of subchondral bone, hyperostotic bone remodeling takes place. In consequence, the bone loses energy absorption capacity, because the pressure and shock absorptive chain is interrupted (Radin and Rose 1986). The distinctive feature of the knee joint is the development of eburnated bone (Fig. 7).

The superficial bone layers then become necrotic, followed by breakage of the border line of bone and microfractures in the subchondral trabeculae (Meachim 1980). The necrotic subchondral bone is replaced by fibrous tissue, developing cysts filled with necrotic bone and cell debris. These cysts are, or were, connected with the subchondral bone marrow (Fig. 8).

On the other hand, cysts or so-called pseudocysts can originate by inflow of synovial fluid into the subchondral bone marrow. The cysts are filled with fibrous or chondroid tissue. In most cases, the connection with the joint space is subsequently closed by callus (Sokoloff 1969), and later differentiation between both types of cysts is impossible.

After the breakage of the subchondral bone, vascularization of the calcified cartilage occurs. Close to the vessels, fibrous or chondroid tissue originates that grows towards the cartilage surface. This vascularization of the cartilage is described as late stage of osteoarthrosis (Mohr 1984).

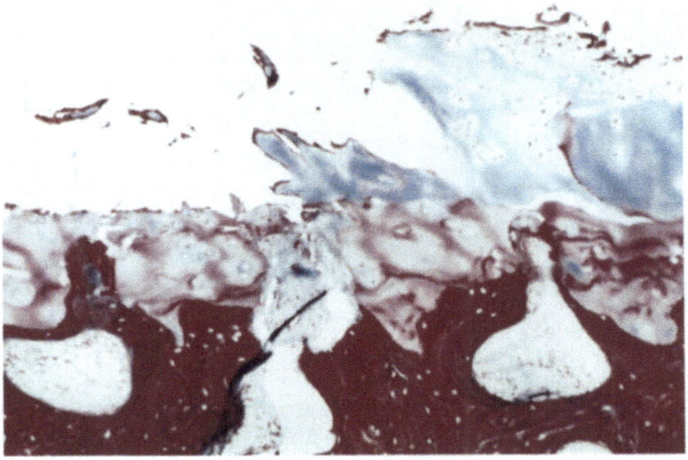

Fig. 6. Lateral femoral condyle in severe varus gonarthrosis. Azan staining, ×100. Hyperostotic subchondral bone, covered only by calcified hyaline cartilage (*left*) or by degenerated noncalcified hyaline cartilage (*right*) with cell cluster formation and cracks up to the tidemark

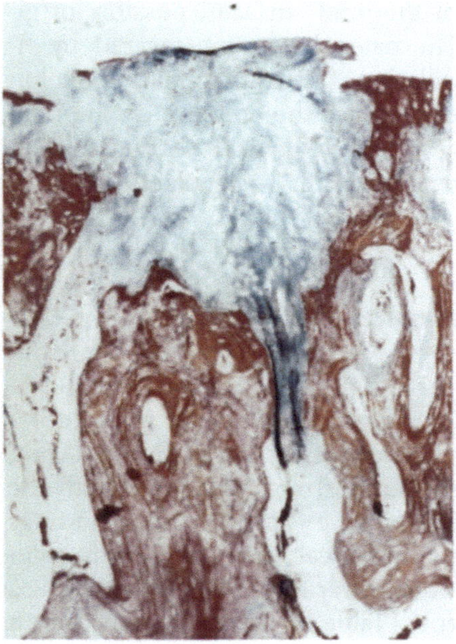

Fig. 7. Medial femoral condyle in severe varus gonarthrosis. Azan staining, ×75. Uncovered hyperostotic subchondral bone, in the center fibrous reparative tissue, which is again a victim of abrasion

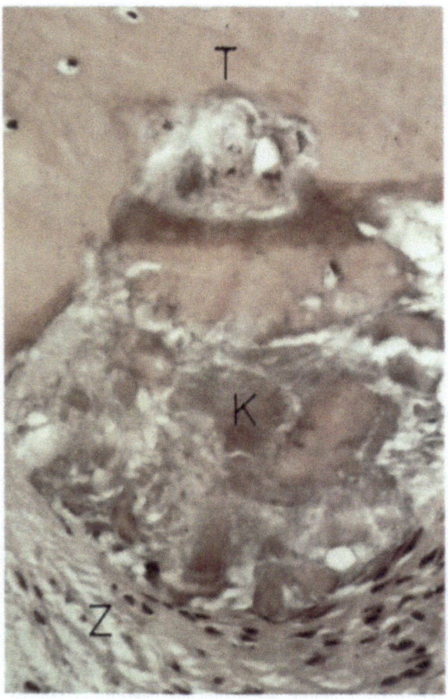

Fig. 8. Medial tibial base plate in severe varus gonarthrosis. Haematoxylin and eosin staining, ×400. Microfracture of subchondral trabecular bone (*T*) with parts of necrotic bone (*K*), below a subchondral cyst (*Z*)

Osteophytes occur at the margins of the joint surfaces, possibly originating by enchondral osteogenesis. The osteophytes are covered by fibrous cartilage, already showing fibrillation (Meachim 1980). Sokoloff (1980) suggested that these osteophytes decrease the pressure on the joint surface by increasing the surface area. In histological sections osteophytes show an osteoporotic bone structure with trabeculae vertical to the joint surface.

Macroscopic, Radiographic, and Histological Findings in Varus Gonarthrosis

In 20 total knee replacements due to varus gonarthrosis the resected osteochondral joint surfaces (Fig. 9) were investigated histologically (Azan, hematoxylin and eosin and Safranin-O staining) and compared with the preoperative radiographic and intraoperative macroscopic findings (Reichel et al. 1997). The radiographic classification (X-rays with anterior-posterior and lateral views) was done separately for the medial and the lateral femoro-tibial compartment (Table 1) according to Wirth (1992). For macroscopic grading, the classification of Brandt et al. (1991) was used (Table 2). Each medial and lateral compartment was graded histologically according to Otte (1969) (Table 3). Based upon the preoperative radiographic findings, the cases were divided into two groups: mod-

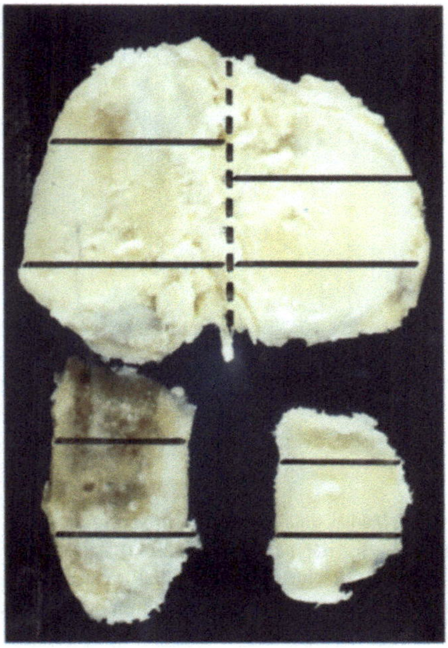

Fig. 9. Tibial base plate (*top*), and medial and lateral distal femoral condyle (*bottom*), resected for total knee replacement due to varus gonarthrosis. Lines demonstrate histologically examined regions

Table 1. Radiographic grading of gonarthrosis (according to Wirth 1992)

Grade	Radiographic findings
I Initial gonarthrosis	– Initial formation of osteophytes on tibial base plate and femoral condyles – Initial narrowing of joint space
II Slight gonarthrosis	– Distinct osteophytes on the tibial base plate – Initial flattening of femoral condyles – Moderate subchondral sclerosis – Slight narrowing of joint space
III Moderate gonarthrosis	– Osteophytes up to 5 mm long – Distinct flattening of femoral condyles – Narrowing of joint space up to one half – Distinct subchondral sclerosis
IV Severe gonarthrosis	– Distinct narrowing up to total loss of joint space – Formation of cysts on femur and tibia up to bony destruction – Osteophytes of more than 5 mm long

Table 2. Macroscopic grading of gonarthrosis (according to Brandt et al. 1991)

Grade	Macroscopic findings
I Initial gonarthrosis	– Loss of cartilage brightness, normal thickness and configuration of cartilage
II Slight gonarthrosis	– Superficial roughness and abrasions of cartilage, but complete cartilage layer
III Moderate gonarthrosis	– Localized cartilage defects with bone shimmering through
IV Severe gonarthrosis	– Visible bony base plate, localized or widespread regenerates of fibrous cartilage

erate (group A) and severe (group B) varus gonarthrosis. The results are shown in Table 4 and Figs. 10 and 11. Even in cases with radiographic and macroscopic grades 1 and 2 lateral changes, the histological sections showed late stages of osteoarthrosis (grades 3 and 4). The lateral femorotibial compartment especially cannot be correctly graded by preoperative X-rays.

Conclusions

Osteoarthrosis of the knee joint leads to an irreversible degeneration of the medial and lateral compartments. In cases of varus gonarthrosis, the involvement of the medial part of the knee is more extensive than of the lateral part. The radiographic and macroscopic gradings show large dif-

Table 3. Histological grading of gonarthrosis (modified according to Otte 1969)

Grade	Histological findings
I Inital gonarthrosis	– Loss of proteoglycans – Necroses of superficial chondrocytes – Reduction of superficial cell density – Superficial horizontal and vertical cracks
II Slight gonarthrosis	– Progressive fibrillations – Clusters of vital chondrocytes – Vertical cracks, exceeding the radius zone – Beginning of cartilage thickness decrease
III Moderate gonarthrosis	– Unmasked collagen fibres – Ingrowth of pannus in the hyaline cartilage (formation of lagoons and cartilage destruction) – Widening of calcified cartilage zone – Duplication of tidemark – Cracks in the tidemark zone – Beginning of subchondral hyperostosis
IV Severe gonarthrosis	– Subchondral hyperostosis – Necroses of osteocytes – Thickness loss until the calcified cartilage – Vascularization of calcified and noncalcified cartilage – Fibrous or chondroid tissue from the subchondral marrow space within the hyaline cartilage – Opening of subchondral bone – Collapse of subchondral bone/formation of pseudocysts

Table 4. Groups of varus gonarthrosis and results of radiographic, macroscopic, and histological grading of medial and lateral compartment

	Group A	Group B
Number of cases	10	10
Varus deviation (from normal femoro-tibial angle of 174°) mean ± SD	7.8 ± 2.8°	14.1 ± 4.3°
Radiographic grading (mean)		
Medial compartment	2.9	1.3
Lateral compartment	4.0	2.7
Macroscopic grading (mean)		
Medial compartment	3.95	2.65
Lateral compartment	4.0	2.65
Histological grading (mean)		
Medial compartment	4.0	3.95
Lateral compartment	4.0	3.95

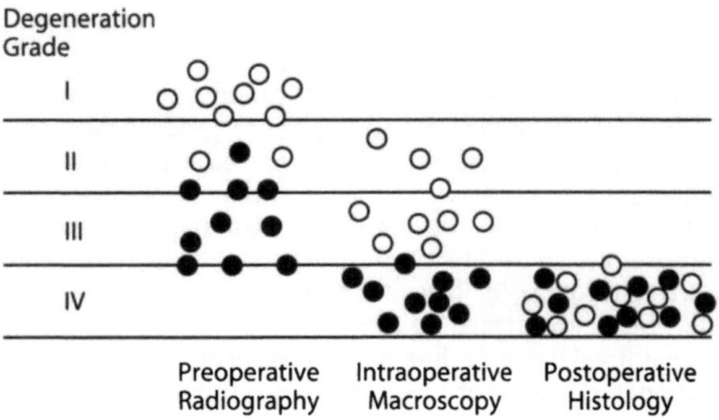

Fig. 10. Comparison of radiographic, macroscopic and histological findings in medial and lateral compartment (group A; *n* = *10*). *Filled circles*, medial compartment; *open circles*, lateral compartment

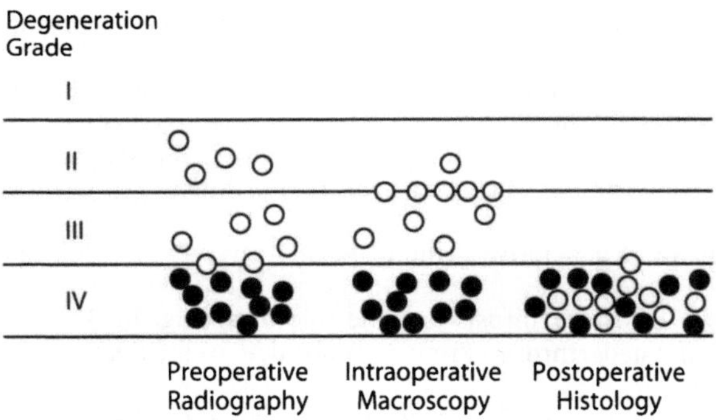

Fig. 11. Comparison of radiographic, macroscopic and histological findings in medial and lateral compartment (group B; *n* = 10). *Filled circles*, medial compartment; *open circles*, lateral compartment

ferences between the medial and the lateral femoro-tibial compartments. Based upon the better condition of the lateral cartilage, high tibial osteotomies in younger patients and unicompartmental knee replacements in older patients are still used in the surgical treatment of varus gonarthrosis. However, histologically the cartilage degeneration of the lateral compartment already shows an irreversible late stage of osteoarthrosis. In our opinion, these findings have to be taken into consideration, especially for patients with varus gonarthrosis younger than 50 years of age. If the varus gonarthrosis is too severe for a joint preserving procedure such as a high tibial osteotomy, in younger patients we prefer to do a total knee replacement rather than a unicompartmental knee replacement.

References

Brandt KD, Fife RS, Braunstein EM, Katz B (1991) Radiographic grading of the severity of knee osteoarthritis: relation of the Kellgren and Lawrence grade based on joint space narrowing, and correlation with arthroscopic evidence of articular cartilage degeneration. Arthritis Rheum 34:1381–1386

Dustmann HO, Puhl W (1978) Das Phänomen der Cluster als pathognomonisches Zeichen der Präarthrose und Arthrose. Z Orthop 116:436

Hackenbroch MH (1992) Periphere Arthrosen. In: Jäger M, Wirth CJ (eds) Praxis der Orthopädie. 2., neubearb. Aufl. Thieme, Stuttgart, pp 596–603

Meachim G (1980) Ways of cartilage breakdown in human and experimental osteoarthrosis. In: Nuki G (ed) The etiopathogenesis of osteoarthrosis. Pitman, Tunbridge Wells, Kent, pp 16–28

Mohr W (1984) Arthrosis deformans. In: Doerr W, Seifert G (eds) Spezielle pathologische Anatomie, Bd. 18/1. Springer, Berlin Heidelberg New York, pp 257–372

Otte P (1969) Die konservative Behandlung der Hüft- und Kniearthrose und ihre Gefahren. Dt Med J 20:604–609

Otte P (1974) Pathophysiologische Grundlagen präarthrotischer Faktoren. Z Orthop 112:541–547

Radin EL, Rose RM (1986) Role of subchondral bone in the initiation and progression of cartilage damage. Clin Orthop 213:34–40

Reichel H, Hein M, Hein W (1997) Vergleich des röntgenologischen, makroskopischen und histologischen Schädigungsgrades bei der Varusgonarthrose. Z Orthop 135:124–130

Sokoloff L (1969) The biology of degenerative joint disease. University of Chicago Press, Chicago

Sokoloff L (1980) The pathology of osteoarthrosis and the role of ageing. In: Nuki G (ed) The aetiopathogenesis of osteoarthrosis. Pitman, Tunbridge Wells, Kent, pp 1–15

Stiller D (1982) Die Pathologie der Arthrose. Zbl allg Path Path Anat 126:425–446

von der Mark K (1986) Differentiation, modulation, and dedifferentiation of chondrocytes. Rheumatology 10:272–315

Wirth CJ (1992) Kniegelenk. In: Jäger M, Wirth CJ (eds) Praxis der Orthopädie. 2., neubearb. Aufl. Thieme, Stuttgart, pp 927–969

Arthroscopic Management of Degenerative Joint Disease

D. J. Ogilvie-Harris and C.-H. Choi

Introduction

Nearly 70% of the population over 65 years of age demonstrate radiographic evidence of osteoarthritis. Since the introduction of arthroscopy, attempts have been made to treat the damaged articular cartilage or to achieve regeneration. Even though articular cartilage appears to have some regenerative capacity, restoration of articular surfaces is very difficult. No technique has been completely successful in achieving normal hyaline cartilage. More recently, the biochemical and biomechanical understanding of articular cartilage has facilitated cartilage cell transplantation, but more studies are in progress for verification of effects and generalized use.

Arthroscopic lavage, arthroscopic abrasion and debridement have had a basic role in the treatment of knee osteoarthritis. Although these techniques provide temporary relief of symptoms and there are many controversies, arthroscopic surgeons should have knowledge of these techniques. These operations provide symptom relief primarily and may delay the secondary definite procedures. These techniques are simple, not time consuming and economic with low morbidity.

The arthroscopic treatment for degenerative arthritis can be divided into simple lavage, debridement and abrasion arthroplasty.

Arthroscopic Lavage

Arthroscopic lavage of the osteoarthritic knee joint provides temporary and short-term relief of symptoms. Although several studies showed favorable results with this technique, not all surgeons consider arthroscopic lavage to be an adequate or optimal surgery in osteoarthritis (Table 1).

Jackson et al. (1986) compared lavage to debridement and reported 68% of patients had permanent improvement with debridement compared with 45% permanent improvement with lavage alone. In a controlled study, Livesley et al. (1991) investigated the hypothesis that joint lavage often provides symptomatic relief for painful osteoarthritis of the

Author	Year	Number of cases	Follow-up (months)	Excellent/ good (%)	Fair/poor (%)
Jackson	1986		39	45	55
Chang	1993	14	12	58	42
Edelson	1995	21	24	81	19
Hubbard	1996	26	52	11[a]	89[a]

[a] Results evaluated with number of pain-free knees.

knee. They found that there was better relief of pain in the lavage group compared to the physiotherapy group and the effect was present at 1 year. They concluded that joint lavage is effective in the management of painful osteoarthritis of the knee. Gibson et al. (1992) measured the effect of arthroscopic lavage and debridement of the osteoarthritis knee by comparing objective measurements of thigh muscle function before and after operation, and they found that there was some improvement in quadriceps isokinetic torque at 6 and 12 weeks after joint lavage but not after debridement. Chang et al. (1993) carried out a controlled study to compare arthroscopic surgery and closed needle joint lavage for patients with non-end-stage osteoarthritis of the knee. They found that after 1 year, 44% of subjects who underwent arthroscopy reported improvement and 58% of subjects who underwent joint lavage improved. They concluded that the search for and removal of soft tissue abnormalities via arthroscopic surgery did not appear justified for all patients who failed to respond to conservative therapy. It may be beneficial for certain subgroups, such as those with clear-cut mechanical symptoms. Edelson et al. (1995) reported a good or excellent results in 17 (81%) of 21 knees with symptomatic osteoarthritis, which underwent washout with lactated Ringer's solution and they confirmed the value of a fluid washout in an arthritic knee for some patients. They used 3 l of fluid running through the knee by using varying inflow and outflow. In a prospective randomized trial, Hubbard (1996) treated 76 knees with isolated degenerative changes in the medial femoral condyle (grades 3 or 4) by either arthroscopic debridement (40) or wash out (36). He found that 19 of a total of 32 survivors in the debridement group and three of the 26 in the washout group were still free from pain. He concluded that arthroscopic debridement appears to be the better treatment, leaving over half the patients free from pain after 5 years.

Arthroscopic Debridement

Arthroscopic debridement is a valuable procedure in the management of osteoarthritis of the knee joint (Table 2). Although palliative in nature, in many instances it yields long-term relief in the low demand knee. It is especially valuable in young individuals who have not yet reached the ideal age for reconstruction. The procedure is a demanding one, requiring considerable arthroscopic skills. Sclerotic lesions, synovitis, loose bodies, osteophytes, chondromalacia, and degenerative tears of meniscii are encountered often in various combinations and must be addressed judiciously and completely. The procedure simplifies rehabilitation, and the risk/benefit ration is very favorable compared to open procedures (Schonholtz et al. 1989).

Sprague reported arthroscopic debridement as a treatment option for unicompartmental osteoarthritis in 1981. He reviewed 68 cases with degenerative arthritis treated with arthroscopic debridement and obtained 74% good results (defined as one in which the patient reported the knee was improved and more functional than before surgery at 14 months of follow up). The extent of arthritis, however, was not correlated clinically or roentgenographically with success rates. Salisbury et al. (1985) reviewed 52 patients with severe degenerative joint disease of the knees treated by arthroscopic debridement and suggested that the results of ar-

Table 2. Results of arthroscopic debridement studies

Author	Year	Number of cases	Follow-up (months)	Excellent/ good (%)	Fair/poor (%)
Sprague	1981	69	14	74	26
Shahriaree	1982	172	84	76	24
Richards	1984	21	40	81	19
Jackson	1986		39	68	32
Bert	1989	67	60	66	34
Baumgaertner	1990	49	33	52	48
Timoney	1990	111	51	45	55
Aichroth	1991	254	44	75	25
Gross	1991	43	24	72	38
Ogilvie-Harris	1991	103[a]	52	66	34
		135[b]	43	41	59
Rand	1991	131	60	67	33
McLaren	1991	171	25	65	35
Su	1995	14	30–132	56	44
Hubbard	1996	32	60	59	41
Linschoten	1997	56	49	68	32

[a] Debridement results for degenerative arthritis involving one compartment.
[b] Debridement results for degenerative arthritis involving two compartments.
[c] Percentage for pain free.

throscopic debridement on normally aligned degenerative knees are encouraging. They also concluded that a combination of arthroscopic debridement and high tibial osteotomy could be an appealing alternative to total knee arthroplasty in the young patients. Patients with varus angular deformity in the degenerative knee had poor results and should be excluded from consideration for arthroscopic debridement. Jackson et al. (1986) reported 68% improved with arthroscopic debridement at 39 months follow up. Baumgaertner et al. (1990) reported good or excellent results in 49 osteoarthritic knees after arthroscopic debridement and postulated that age, weight, compartment location of arthritis, and presurgical range of motion did not affect surgical results. They also found symptoms of long duration, arthritic severity as evidenced by roentgenograms, and malalignment predicted poor results, and conversely, shorter duration of symptoms, mechanical symptoms, mild to moderate roentgenographic changes and crystal deposition correlated with improved results. Timoney et al. (1990) found that the overall result was good in 45% in 111 knees at the follow up of 51 months after arthroscopic debridement. However, they reported that arthroscopic debridement offered measurable relief for 63% of patients for a significant period of time, and 74% of the patients felt the procedure had been beneficial. In a retrospective study undertaken for evaluation arthroscopic debridement, Gross et al. (1991) obtained 72 good results at follow up of 24 months in 43 knees and suggested that preoperative clinical status, severity of degenerative changes, and number of pathologic entities encountered at the time of surgery correlated with the results of treatment. Aichroth et al. (1991) reported that 75% had minimal discomfort and improved function and 85% were satisfied with the treatment at follow-up of 44 months in 254 patients. He obtained better results in the cases with less radiographic changes, less severe involvement of articular cartilage at operation and younger age. They also found that only 14% had a subsequent operation after an average period of 4 years. Rand (1991) reported 80% improvement at 1 year follow up and 67% improvement at 5 years in 131 patients and postulated that arthroscopic debridement has beneficial effects compared to abrasion arthroplasty. McLaren et al. (1991) reviewed 171 patients with osteoarthrosis of the knee treated with arthroscopic debridement and found excellent control of pain in only 38%, improved function in 22% and subsequent surgical procedures in 12% at an average follow-up of 25 months. They did not identify factors that correlated with the outcome, including the extent of degenerative changes, of debridement and patient profiles. They postulated that arthroscopic debridement is a temporizing procedure with good patient satisfaction. Linschoten and Johnson (1997) analyzed 56 patients who had degenerative arthritis and were treated with arthroscopic debridement and obtained good results in 38 (68%) at an average follow-up of 49 months. They suggested that the presence of severe (grade IV) chondromalacia was associated with subsequent surgery and when the medial compartment was involved, the likelihood of a poor outcome increased significantly. In prospective, randomized and placebo-controlled trial, Moseley et al. (1996) evaluated the effects of arthroscopic debridement and lavage in ten patients. Even though the number of patients was too small to be statistically significant, they suggested that there might be a significant placebo effect for arthroscopic treatment of osteoarthritis of the knee.

Abrasion Arthroplasty

Pridie originated the concept of abrasion arthroplasty through eburnated bone to stimulate reparative cartilage formation from drilling technique in 1959. He described fibrous-like reparative cartilage filling and covering one-quarter inch cortical drill holes through the femoral condyle and reported on 62 knees in 60 patients. Of 62 patients, 46 felt their operation was a success and stated that they would have the operation again under similar circumstances. Salter et al. (1980) provided the basic science showing that 2 mm holes drilled into cancellous bone led to fibrocartilaginous repair in animals when continuous passive motion was employed.

Johnson (1986) advocated abrading only the areas of exposed bone that were already denuded of hyaline cartilage (Table 3). He postulated that the depth of debridement, felt to be critical, should be limited to 1–2 mm into the intracortical layer to expose vascularity providing a tissue bed for blood clot attachment. He felt that deeper abrasion into the sub-

Table 3. Results of arthroscopic abrasion studies

Author	Year	Number of cases	Follow-up (months)	Excellent/ good (%)	Fair/poor (%)
Richards	1984	22	25	80	20
Friedman	1984	73		60	40
Johnson	1986		24	77	23
Bert	1989	59	60	51	49
Ogilvie-Harris	1991	32	49	53	47
Rand	1991	28	45	50	50
Singh	1991	52	3–27	51	49
Haspl	1995	21	12–60	90	10
Su	1995	18[a]	30–132	57	43
Steadman	1998	35[b]	24–288	75	25

[a] Treated with arthroscopic drilling.
[b] Treated with microfracture.

chondral layer produced poor results. He also recommended this procedure primarily for patients with normal mechanical alignment, good range of motion and low activity demands. Contraindications included varus angulation of greater than 10° or valgus angulation greater than 15° as well as evidence of inflammatory joint disease. Singh et al. (1991) reported that the 51% of patients with degenerative arthritis was improved with abrasion arthroplasty and the results were better in the older age group and in those without significant deformity. They found also that there was improvement in 74% of patients with normal alignment. Friedman et al. (1984) reported that 60% of patients who were treated with abrasion arthroplasty in degenerative arthritis and the results were best in patients younger than 40 years of age. Akizuki et al. (1997) investigated whether or not abrasion arthroplasty promotes cartilage regeneration in osteoarthritis knee and found a significant high incidence of grade II healing in the osteotomy with abrasion group compared to osteotomy group. However, they did not find difference in clinical outcome at 2–9 years postoperatively between two groups. Miller at al. (1986) reported that four of five patients who had idiopathic medial femoral condyle osteonecrosis, were rated good after arthroscopic debridement and abrasion arthroplasty. In a study comparing abrasion arthroplasty and subchondral drilling in the rabbit, Menche et al. (1996) found that subchondral drilling may result in a longer lived repair than abrasion arthroplasty after histologic examination at 6 weeks. Goldman et al. (1997) postulated that abrasion arthroplasty and the Pridie procedure do not appear to offer any additional benefit to arthroscopic debridement alone and arthroscopic debridement is the preferred procedure to abrasion arthroplasty. Rand and Ritts (1989) treated with abrasion arthroplasty in 8 patients with persistent pain after upper tibial osteotomy and correction of malalignment and concluded that abrasion arthroplasty is not a satisfactory salvage for a failed upper tibial osteotomy. Rand (1991) compared arthroscopic partial meniscectomy with limited debridement compared to arthroscopic abrasion arthroplasty in patients with osteoarthritis. All patients had grade III and IV chondromalacia change. Group I (131 patients) was treated with arthroscopic meniscectomy and debridement and group II (28 patients) was treated with abrasion arthroplasty. He found that 50% of the abrasion group subsequently underwent a total knee arthroplasty for salvage at a mean of 3 years following the abrasion procedure and, concluded that abrasion arthroplasty appears to offer little benefit over partial meniscectomy and debridement at 3.6 years follow up. In a comparative study abrasion arthroplasty with arthroscopic debridement, Bert and Maschka (1989) reported that 66% had good to excellent results in 67 patients of arthroscopic debridement, the other hand, 51% had good to excellent results in 59 patients of abrasion arthroplasty at a mean follow up time of 60 months.

One must conclude that the literature overall shows little benefit to the patient in abrasion arthroplasty compared with arthroscopic debridement alone. On an intellectual level, it would seem to be of benefit to knees in which there were localized full thickness defects of articular cartilage. This has been confirmed recently by Steadman. He reported his results using the microfracture technique incorporating abrasion arthroplasty and debridement at the 65th Annual Meeting of the American Academy of Orthopaedic Surgeons (1998). He followed 235 patients for 2–12 years. At 3 years 75% of patients had improved, 19% unchanged, and 6% were worse. 66% had improved ability to do strenuous work, 59% did strenuous sports and the activity of daily living improved in 68%. The rates of improvement remained steady without deterioration for up to 10 years. A total of 5% of patients had secondary procedures by 4 years, and 8% by 7 years.

Our Experience and Recommendations

We initially published our results in 1991. Since then we have completed a 5-year review on the same group of patients. Our results demonstrate that good results can be obtained with reasonable long-term duration (Table 4). Out of a total 551 arthroscopic procedures for degenerative arthritis of the knee, 441 were studied at 2–10 years following their procedure. In total, 68% of patients had at least 2 years or more relief of pain and symptoms; 53% were still good at follow-up of 6 years. The best results were obtained after resection of an unstable flap tear of a meniscus in association with mild degenerative arthritis. The worst results were obtained in patients with bicondylar disease and in the presence of chondrocalcinosis. The results were much better in the normally aligned knee; the valgus knee did worst. Repeated arthroscopic procedures have a much lower success rate (Table 5).

We recommend arthroscopic debridement as the primary surgical treatment for the following patients:

Table 4. Results by procedure

	Number	Good at 2 years	Good at 5 years
Debride 1 compartment	103	84 (82%)	68 (66%)
Debride 2 compartments	135	78 (58%)	52 (39%)
Abrasion	32	18 (56%)	15 (46%)
Meniscectomy	18	15 (83%)	12 (66%)
Meniscectomy and debridement	149	102 (68%)	87 (58%)

Table 5. Results by previous operations

Arthroscopy	Number	Good at 2 years	Good at 5 years
First	334	71%	57%
Second	107	61%	37%
Third	50	56%	32%
Fourth or more	57	37%	27%

1. Significant mechanical symptoms, such as locking, pain on walking, giving out
2. Mild to moderate osteoarthritic changes on X-ray with some preservation of the joint space on the tunnel views
3. Failed conservative treatment, such as nonsteroid antiinflamatory drugs, cortisone or hyaluronic injections, physiotherapy with an exercise program (e.g "knee school")
4. Persistent pain limiting important aspects of the patient's life
5. Reasonable alignment of the knee
6. Ligamentous stability.

We feel it is contraindicated in the following patients:

1. Inflammatory arthritis such as rheumatoid arthritis
2. Significant varus or valgus, especially with ligament pseudolaxity
3. Severe loss of joint space on X-ray with bone on bone contact
4. Severe chondrocalcinosis
5. Previous failed arthroscopic debridement – second and subsequent arthroscopic debridements are much less successful. If the symptomatic relief has been less than 2 years, we regard that as failure (Table 6).

We would offer arthroscopic abrasion by any of the accepted techniques to the following:

1. Patients with failed arthroscopic debridement, where the pathology was clearly a localized full thickness defect of up to one half of one femoral condyle
2. Minimal loss of joint space on X-ray
3. No ligamentous laxity
4. No significant malalignment (an abnormal alignment could be corrected concurrently with an osteotomy)
5. Osteochondritis dissecans, when the lesion was not repairable.

Further cartilage replacement procedures such as autologous transfers, or autologous chondrocyte transplantation would only be offered to patients when the above procedures were unsuccessful, providing they met the other criteria for the surgery.

Table 6. Predictors for success and failure after arthroscopic lavage, arthroscopic debridement and arthroscopic abrasion in the literature

Good predictors	Bad predictors
Old age group	Young age group
Mechanical symptoms	Inflammatory symptoms
Short symptom duration	Long symptom duration
Minimal sign of degeneration	Severe chondromalacia
Normal limb alignment	Malalignment
Crystal deposition	Medial compartment involvement

References

Aichroth PM, Patel DV, Moyes ST (1991) A prospective review of arthroscopic debridement for degenerative joint disease of the knee. Int Orthop 15:351–355

Akizuki S, Yasukawa Y, Takizawa T (1997) Does arthroscopic abrasion arthroplasty promote cartilage regeneration in osteoarthritic knees with eburnation? A prospective study of high tibial osteotomy with abrasion arthroplasty versus high tibial osteotomy alone. Arthroscopy 13:9–17

Baumgaertner MR, Cannon WD Jr, Vittori JM, Schmidt ES, Mauere RC (1990) Arthroscopic debridement of the arthritic knee. Clin Orthop 253:197–202

Bert JM (1993) Role of abrasion arthroplasty and debridement in the management of osteoarthritis of the knee. Rheum Dis Clin North Am 19:725–739

Bert JM, Maschka K (1989) The arthroscopic treatment of unicompartmental gonarthrosis: a five year follow-up study of abrasion arthroplasty plus arthroscopic debridement and arthroscopic debridement alone. Arthroscopy 5:25–32

Chang RW, Falconer J, Stulberg SD, Arnold WJ, Manheim LM, Dyer AR (1993) A randomized, controlled trial of arthroscopic surgery versus closed-needle joint lavage for patients with osteoarthritis of the knee. Arthritis Rheum 36:289–296

Edelson R, Burk RT, Bloebaum RD (1995) Short-term effects of knee washout for osteoarthritis. Am J Sports Med 23:345–349

Friedman MJ, Berasi, CC, Fox JM, Del Pisso W, Snyder SJ, Ferkel RD (1984) Preliminary results with abrasion arthroplasty in the osteoarthritic knee. Clin Orthop 182:200–205

Gibson JN, White MD, Chapman VM, Strachan RK (1992) Arthroscopic lavage and debridement for osteoarthritis of the knee. J Bone Joint Surg 74B:534–537

Goldman RT, Scuderi GR, Kelly MA (1997) Arthroscopic treatment of the degenerative knee in older athletes. Clin Sports Med 16:51–68

Gross DE, Brenner SL, Estormes I, Gross ML (1991) The arthroscopic treatment of degenerative joint disease in the knee. J Orthop 14:1317–1321

Haspl M, Pecina M (1995) Treatment of gonarthrosis with arthroscopic abrasion. Leduc Vjesn 117:236–240

Hubbard MJ (1996) Articular debridement versus washout for degeneration of the medial femoral condyle. A five-year study. J Bone Joint Surg 78B:217–219

Jackson RW, Silver R, Marans H (1986) The arthroscopic treatment of degenerative joint disease. Arthroscopy 2:114–119

Johnson LL (1986) Arthroscopic abrasion arthroplasty historical and pathologic perspective: present status. Arthroscopy 2:54–69

Linschoten NJ, Johnson CA (1997) Arthroscopic debridement of knee joint arthritis: effect of advancing articular degeneration. J South Orthop Assoc 6:25–36

Livesley PJ, Doherty M, Needoff M, Moulton A (1991) Arthroscopic lavage of osteoarthritic knee. J Bone Joint Surg 73B:922–926
McLaren AC, Blokker CP, Fowler PJ, Roth JN, Rock MG (1991) Arthroscopic debridement of the knee for osteoarthrosis. Can J Surg 34:595–598
Menche DS, Frenkel SR, Blair B, Watnik NF, Toolan BC, Yaghuobian RS, Pitman MI (1996) A comparison of abrasion burr arthroplasty and subchondral drilling in the treatment of full-thickness cartilage lesions in the rabbit. Arthroscopy 12:280–286
Miller GK, Maylahn DJ, Drennan DB (1986) The treatment of idiopathic osteonecrosis of the medial femoral condyle with arthroscopic debridement. Arthroscopy 2:21–29
Moseley JB Jr, Wray NP, Kuykendall D, Willis K, Landon G (1996) Arthroscopic treatment of osteoarthritis of the knee: a prospective, randomized, placebo-controlled trial. Results of a pilot study. Am J Sports Med 24:28–34
Ogilvie-Harris DJ, Fitsialos DP (1991) Arthroscopic management of the degenerative knee. Arthroscopy 7:151–157
Pridie KH (1959) A method of resurfacing osteoarthritic knee joints. J Bone Joint Surg 41B:618–624
Rand JA (1991) Role of arthroscopy in osteoarthritis of the knee. Arthroscopy 7:358–363
Rand JA, Ritts GD (1989) Abrasion arthroplasty as a salvage for failed upper tibial osteotomy. J Arthroplasty 4 [Suppl]:45–48
Richards RN, Lonergen RP (1984) Arthroscopic surgery for relief of pain in the osteoarthritic knee. Orthopedics 7:1705–1721
Salisbury RB, Nottage WM, Gardner V (1985) The effect of alignment on results in arthroscopic debridement of the degenerative knee. Clin Orthop 198:268–272
Salter R, Simmonds D, Malcolm B et al. (1980) The biological effect of continuous passive motion on the healing of full thickness defects in articular cartilage. J Bone Joint Surg 62A:1232–1251
Schonholtz GJ (1989) Arthroscopic debridement of the knee joint. Orthop Clin North Am 20:257–263
Shahriaree H, O'Connor RF, Nottage W (1982) Seven years follow-up arthroscopic debridement of the degenerative knee. Field of View 1:1–9
Singh S, Lee CC, Tay BK (1991) Results of arthroscopic abrasion arthroplasty in osteoarthritis of the knee joint. Singapore Med J 32:34–37
Sprague NF III (1981) Arthroscopic debridement for degenerative knee joint disease. Clin Orthop 160:118–123
Steadman JR (1998) Presented at the American Academy of Orthopaedic Surgery
Su JY, Chang JK, Lu YM, Lin SY (1995) Arthroscopic debridement for osteoarthritis of the knee: a seven years follow-up study. Kao Hsiung I Hsueh Ko Hsueh Tsa Chih 11:667–672
Timoney JM, Kneisl JS, Barrack RL, Alexander AH (1990) Arthroscopy update 6. Arthroscopy in the osteoarthritic knee. Long-term follow-up. Orthop Rev 19:376–379

Arthroscopic and Open Techniques for Transplantation of Osteochondral Autografts and Allografts in Different Joints

A. B. Imhoff, G. M. Oettl, P. Schöttle, J. Agneskirchner, and A. Burkart

Introduction

A chondral/osteochondral defect involving the articular surface of a joint is still a therapeutic problem. The goal of articular cartilage repair is restoration of cartilage congruity, accomplishing full pain-free range of motion and elimination of cartilage deterioration (Bobic 1996; Imhoff and Öttl 1997; Öttl et al. 1997). There are a variety of methods of treatment. Current treatments are: debridement and drilling, picking or abrasion of the subchondral bone (Johnson 1991; Rodrigo et al. 1994; Tippet 1996), fresh osteochondral allografts (Garret 1997; Gross 1997), periosteal or perichondral grafting (Homminga et al. 1990; Lorentzon 1996), periosteal grafting with chondrocyte transplant (Brittberg et al. 1994; Peterson 1997) and joint replacement. The use of autologous grafts was first reported by Wagner and Müller in 1964 (Müller 1978; Wagner 1964). The use of cylindrical autograft plugs was described by Bobic (1996) (osteochondral autograft transfer system, OATS) and Hangody et al. (1996) (mosaicplasty). Although originally developed for the treatment of focal chondral and osteochondral defects of the weight-bearing surfaces of the femur, it can also be used on the patella, tibia, elbow, talar dome, shoulder and hip.

Indications and Patient Selection Criteria

Osteochondral autograft transplantation is an option for patients with a symptomatic unipolar focal chondral or osteochondral defect (OCD) or focal osteonecrosis but no osteoarthrosis. Tibiofemoral or patellofemoral malalignment and/or functional instability (anterior or posterior cruciate ligament injuries) must be managed concurrently or prior to the chondral injury (Bobic 1996; Hangody et al. 1996).

Surgical Technique

The aim is to harvest autogenous osteochondral cylindrical plugs with healthy cartilage from a non-weight-bearing zone of the knee joint and transfer it to the damaged area. The technique can be done arthroscopically or as an open procedure depending on the location and the size of the osteochondral defect and also of the harvest site. The cylindrical grafts can range in size from 5 mm to 15 mm in diameter. Using special instruments one can harvest the graft at a uniform diameter and depth (Fig. 1). The chondral lesion is inspected arthroscopically, the extent of the defect is determined and the decision to transfer one or more cylinders must be made. One can use special sizers for this purpose. If magnetic resonance imaging (MRI) is available, the size of the defect can be determined preoperatively. Then the decision of whether an arthroscopic or open procedure is needed follows. In an open procedure, our surgical approach is a mini-arthrotomy or direct mid-line allowing access for the harvesting and insertion of the osteochondral plugs. If necessary, an osteotomy for the additional treatment of varus or valgus deformity is also carried out. The arthroscopic technique is adjusted by changing the portal and/or knee flexion angle in order to locate the defect and to ensure a precise angle of fit on the articular cartilage surface. We use special thin-walled cutting tubes in different diameters from 5 to 15 mm to harvest the cylindrical bone plugs. The recipient site is prepared by removing a bone core 1 mm less in diameter than the donor site. Then the donor autograft plug will press fit into the recipient tunnel with firm fixation (Fig. 2).

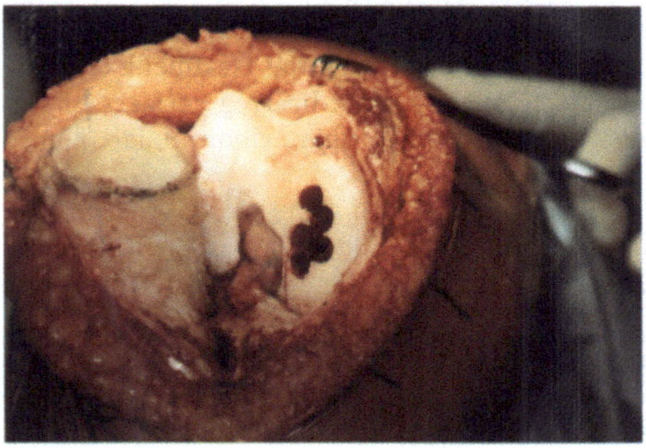

Fig. 1. In an open procedure our surgical approach is a mini-arthrotomy or direct mid-line allowing access for the harvesting and insertion of the osteochondral plugs. We use special thin-walled cutting tubes in different diameters from 5 to 15 mm to harvest the cylindrical bone plugs

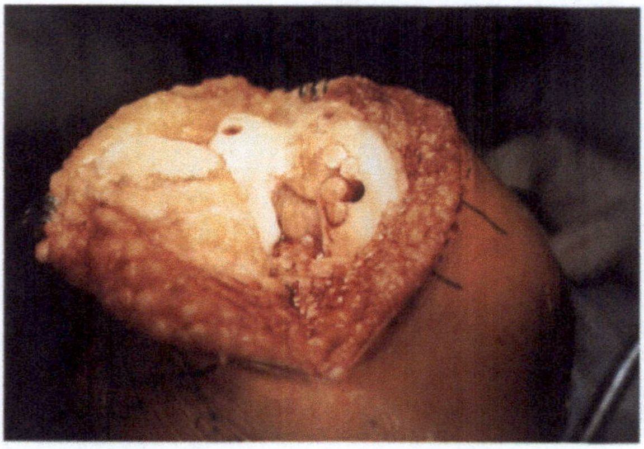

Fig. 2. After donor plug harvesting the overall length can be measured and matched with the tunnel length of the recipient site. After donor core insertion depth control and final core seating the donor plug is inserted, press fit, and finally seated flush with surrounding cartilage

Usually the length of the removed recipient bone core is about 15 mm. After smoothly removing the core, the correct depth of the recipient tunnel is measured. The preferred donor site is the non-weight bearing zone of the ipsilateral femoral condyle in the anterior proximal lateral area. The lateral intercondylar notch is an alternative donor zone. To reach the former, a standard lateral portal with the knee flexed about 30° is made. Sometimes donor and recipient sites can be reached through one portal. After donor plug harvesting the overall length can be measured and matched with the tunnel length of the recipient site. After donor core depth control and final core seating, the donor plug is inserted 'press fit' and finally seated flush with surrounding cartilage (Fig. 3). The graft should fit perfectly in terms of surface contour and height with firm fixation. High and low spots are deleterious. In case of multiple osteochondral transfers each transfer should be finished completely, in order to place subsequent donor plugs directly adjacent to previously inserted bone plugs (Fig. 4). Donor tunnels are either grafted with cancellous bone from the defect or left open. Postoperative management includes pain control, antibiotics and deep vein thrombosis prophylaxis. We mobilized the knee with continuous passive motion to maximize cartilage nutrition. Then, the patients were non-weight-bearing for 6–8 weeks, and protected weight-bearing for 12 weeks, with full range of motion and isometric exercises throughout.

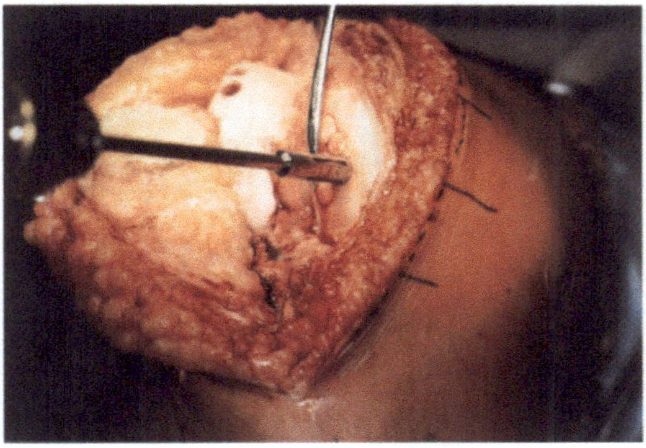

Fig. 3. In multiple osteochondral transfers each transfer should be finished in order to place subsequent donor plugs directly adjacent to previously inserted bone plugs

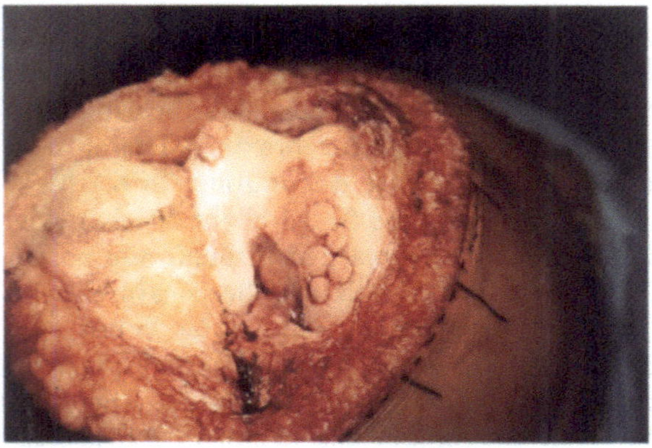

Fig. 4. The graft should be orthotop fitting perfectly in terms of surface contour and height with firm fixation. High and low spots are deleterious

Additional Interventions

The autologous graft should not be placed in a compartment that is bearing more than physiological load. In case of varus or valgus deformity, an osteotomy can be performed simultaneously. In the case of functional anterior instability an ACL-repair is indicated.

Technique of Two-Joint Procedure

Two-joint procedure involves harvesting osteochondral bone plugs from the knee, to be implanted in the ankle or other joints. For treatment for OCD of the talar dome using an open technique, the focal lesions should be 10 mm or greater in diameter. The grafts are harvested either arthroscopically or from an open incision from the medial or lateral anterior proximal femoral condyle. To expose the medial talar dome, often a medial malleolus osteotomy is necessary. Sometime a partial anterior resection of the malleolus is sufficient. To access the lateral dome, division of the anterior talofibular ligament is necessary. For osteochondral transfer to the patella or the elbow an open procedure is necessary.

Results

Operative management and early results of osteochondral cylindrical autograft plugs in the femoral condyle, patella, elbow and talar dome have been reviewed. Since 1996, 80 patients (37 female, 43 male), mean age 31 years (17–59), with osteochondral defects of 1.5–7 cm^2 at the femoral condyle (36 patients), 1–3 cm^2 at the patella (12 patients), 1–3 cm^2 at the talus (21 patients) and 2 cm^2 at the elbow (three patients) and at the shoulder joint (two patients) were treated with transplantation of cylindrical autograft plugs in OATS-technique from the non-weight-bearing zone of the femoral condyle. One to six plugs of different diameters were inserted for repair of the cartilage defect. Six patients had a combined high tibial osteotomy (HTO) or ACL-repair (twelve patients). Follow-up is 3–20 months (mean 9 months). Patients underwent clinical assessment (OCD Score Bruns-Lysholm) as well as X-ray evaluation and MRI follow up in all cases. In addition, certain cases had a second-look arthroscopy.

Overall, evaluation with the Visual Analog Scale showed twentyfive patients had excellent results, thirtysix good results, while three patients had only fair results. All patients had an improvement in modified Bruns-Lysholm-score mean 35 (10–40) points. X-ray and MRI with (i.v.-Gadolinium) confirmed complete incorporation, vitality of the graft and congruity of the articular cartilage with different tide mark levels of the plugs. Second-look arthroscopy confirmed hardness of the cartilage of the graft. X-rays showed no deterioration of the knee joint, the other treated joints or enlargement of the defect. MRI performed at various stages during the postoperative period indicated progressive signs of filling in of the defects and congruent joint surfaces. We had the following complications; one plug in an unacceptable position, one broken donor plug, one postoperative hematoma and one plug with late sinkage. Four patients developed postsurgical anterior knee pain located at the site of donor plug harvesting but it was temporary.

Discussion

The arthroscopic/open use of autologous osteochondral grafts from the knee is indicated in chondral/osteochondral lesions in diameter from 1 to 3 cm, which cannot be primarily reattached and in osteonecrosis of the femoral condyle, patella, elbow, and talar dome. Autologous osteochondral implanted grafts require violation of subchondral bone and lead to a corresponding defect at the donor site. Marrow cell techniques such as drilling, microfracture or abrasion arthroplasty have no good mid- or long-term results because they typically promote the development of fibrocartilage. Fibrocartilage does not have the biomechanical properties of the hyaline cartilage (Buckwalter et al. 1990; Johnson 1991; Kim et al. 1991; Mitchell and Shepard 1987; Peterson 1997; Rodrigo et al. 1994; Tippet 1996). Other methods using perichondral and periosteal grafts are described, but these techniques are limited by the amount of tissue available and they have the tendency toward ossification of the repair tissue. A new alternative is autologous chondrocyte implantation (Homminga et al. 1990; Lorentzon 1996). Osteochondral allografts have the risk of viral transmission of disease and low chondrocyte viability, in addition to removal of host bone for implantation. Gross (1997) followed 123 patients (1972–1992) with fresh osteochondral allograft for osteochondral defects of the knee and found 95% success rate at 5 years, 71% at 10 years and 66% at 20 years. Lateral patella facet autografts for repair of large osteochondral defects was described by Outerbridge et al. (1995). They reported on ten patients with an average follow-up of 6.5 years (range, 4–9). All ten patients were satisfied with their results. Yamashita et al. (1985) reported on the transplantation of an autogenic osteochondral graft for osteochondritis dissecans. Two patients with a follow-up of 2 years were asymptomatic. Matsusue et al. (1993) published a case report of arthroscopic repair of a 15 mm-defect using three osteochondral plugs derived from the lateral intercondylar notch during ACL reconstruction. Second-look arthroscopy 2 years after the graft, showed the original defect to be completely covered with chondral tissue. Hangody et al. (1996) reported on 52 patients with autologous osteochondral mosaic-like graft technique for replacing weight-bearing cartilage defects. Histology in eight cases showed hyaline-like gliding surfaces. The HSS score was 82.5 (65–100) postoperatively. He had no reported complications related to the non-weight-bearing donor sites and follow-up arthroscopy of these sites have noted the donor holes filled in with cancelous bone and fibrocartilage. Bobic (1996) reported on 12 cases of arthroscopic osteochondral transplantation of lesions 10–22 mm in diameter. Ten of 12 patients had excellent results at 2 years follow-up. Transfer of the posterior condyle of the femoral condyle has to be considered as a treatment option of very large osteochondral defects (Imhoff and Öttl 1997). Autogenous transplantation of osteochondral plugs requires precise and careful surgery. Each transplanted plug has to be placed at the correct height and inclination as the surrounding surfaces. If it is slightly too low, even by only 0.5 mm, the plug will not have normal articular pressure and will not carry normal articular load and may predispose to late degradation. If it is too high, then it will take an unfairly large part of the joint load and this may lead to loss of the surface of the plug, and perhaps damage to the opposite cartilage counterface on the opposing bone (Amis 1998).

Conclusion

Disadvantages of autogenous osteochondral grafts were the limited supply of autogenous tissue, defects in non-weight-bearing zone with temporary anterior knee pain and a long rehabilitation. Advantages include no disease transmission, high survival rate of the grafted chondrocytes and reliability of autogenous tissue, effective one-step treatment, reconstruction of the congruity of the articular cartilage and the treatment of different joints. Additional interventions such as osteotomy or ACL-repair should be considered.

References

Amis A (1998) Cartilage repair – a bioengineer's viewpoint. International Cartilage Repair Society, Department of Pathology, University of Berne, Newsletter 1:3

Bobic V (1996) Arthroscopic ostechondral autograft transplantation in anterior cruciate ligament reconstruction: a preliminary clinical study. Knee surgery, sports traumatology. Arthroscopy 3:262–264

Brittberg M, Lindahl A, Nilsson A, et al. (1994) Treatment of deep cartilage defects in the knee with autologous chondrocyte implantation. N Engl J Med 331:889–895

Buckwalter JA, Rosenberg LC, Hunziker EB (1990) Articular cartilage: composition, structure, response to injury, and methods of facilitating repair. In: Ewing JW (ed) Articular cartilage and knee joint function: basic science and arthroscopy. Raven Press, New York, pp 19–56

Garret JC (1993) Osteochondral allografts. Instr Course Lect 42:355–358

Gross AE (1997) Long term results of the fresh osteochondral allograft for osteochondral defects of the knee secondary to trauma or osteochondritis dissecans (abstract). AAOS Instructional Course Lecture. Annual AAOS Meeting, San Francisco, p 330

Hangody L, Karpati Z, Udvarhelyi I (1996) Autologous osteochondral mosaic-like graft technique for replacing weight bearing cartilage defects (abstract). 7th ESSKA Congress, Budapest, Hungary, p 99

Homminga GN, Bulstra SK, Bouwmeester PSM, Van der Linden AJ (1990) Perichondrial grafting for cartilage lesions of the knee. J Bone Joint Surg Br 72:1003–1007
Imhoff AB, Oettl G (1997) Autologer Kondylentransfer als Therapiemöglichkeit bei grossen osteochondralen Defekten am Femurkondylus. Deutsch-Oesterreichischer Orthopädenkongress (abstract) (DGOT). Z Orthop 135:A92
Imhoff AB, Burkart A (1998) Knorpelschaden-Knieinstabilität. Das instabile Knie und der Knorpelschaden des Sportlers. Steinkopff, Darmstadt, 189 pp
Imhoff AB, Oettl GM, Burkart A, Traub S (1999) Osteochondrale autologe Transplantation an verschiedenen Gelenken. Orthopäde 28:33–44
Imhoff AB, Burkart A, Oettl GM (1999) Der posteriore Femurkondylentransfer – Erste Erfahrungen mit einer Salvageoperation. Orthopäde 28:45–51
Johnson LL (1991) Arthroscopic abrasion arthroplasty. In: McGinty JB (ed) Operative arthroscopy. Raven Press, New York, pp 341–360
Kim HK, Moran ME, Salter RB (1991) The potential for regeneration of articular cartilage in defects created by chondral shaving and subchondral abrasion. An experimental investigation in rabbits. J Bone Joint Surg 73A:1301–1315
Lorentzon R, Hildingsson Ch, Alfredsson H (1996) Treatment of deep cartilage defects in the knee with periosteum transplantation (abstract). 2nd World Congress on Sports Trauma, 22nd Annual Meeting of the American Orthopedic Society for Sports Medicine, Lake Buenta Vista, Florida, p 475
Matsusue Y, Yamamuro T (1993) Hma H. Case report: Arthroscopic multiple osteochondral transplantation to the chondral defect in the knee associated with cruciate ligament disruption. Arthroscopy 9:318–321
Mitchell N, Shepard N (1987) Effect of patellar shaving in the rabbit. Orthop Res 5:388–392
Mueller W (1978) Osteochondrosis dissecans. In: Hastings DE (ed) Progress in Orthopaedic Surgery, vol 3. Springer, Berlin Heidelberg New York, pp 135–142
Oettl G, Sigel A, Hof N, Schittich I, Imhoff AB, Hipp E (1997) Osteochondrosis dissecans – stadienabhängige Therapie und Verlaufskontrolle mittels MRT – eine prospektive Studie. Deutsch-Österreichischer Orthopädenkongress (abstract) (DGOT) Z Orthop 135:A46
Outerbridge HK, Outerbridge AR, Outerbridge RE (1995) The use of lateral patellar autologous graft for the repair of a large osteochondral defect in the knee. J Bone Joint Surg Am 77:65–72
Peterson L (1996) Chondrocyte transplantation. Surgical technique (abstract). Second World Congress on Sports Trauma/American Orthopedic Society for Sports Medicine (AOSSM) 22nd Annual Meeting, Lake Buena Vista, p 474
Rodrigo JJ, Steadman RJ, Siliman JF, Fulstone HA (1994) Improvement of full-thickness chondral defect healing in the human knee after debridement and microfracture using continuous passive motion. Am J Knee Surg 7:109–116
Tippet JW (1996) Articular cartilage drilling and osteotomy in osteoarthritis of the knee. In: McGinty JB, RB Caspari, RW Jackson, GG Poehling (eds) Operative arthroscopy, 2nd edn. Raven Press, Philadelphia New York, pp 411–426
Wagner H (1964) Operative Behandlung der Osteochondrosis dissecans des Kniegelenkes. Z Orthop 98:333–355
Yamashita F, Sakakida K, Suzu F, Takai S (1985) The transplantation of an autogenic osteochondral fragment for osteochondritis dissecans of the knee. Clin Orthop 201:43–50

Tissue Engineering in Cartilage Repair: In Vitro and In Vivo Experiments on Cell-Seeded Collagen Matrices

S. Nehrer and M. Spector

Introduction

The limited healing response of articular cartilage has been reported for over three centuries (Hunter 1743; Paget 1853). Healing of cartilage depends on blood clot formation as a provisional matrix for cell migration and a subsequent cascade of chondroprogenitor cells derived from adjacent cartilage, underlying marrow, or synovium, which eventually leads to the formation of reparative tissue in the defect (Buckwalter et al. 1988; Johnson 1991). The persistence of full thickness chondral defects in the articular surface (i.e. those that do not initially penetrate the subchondral bone) is multifactorial: the lack of blood supply, insufficient fibrin clot formation at the area of injury (Buckwalter et al. 1988; Mankin et al. 1994), the low mitotic activity of chondrocytes, inhibition of synovial cell attachment (Langer and Gross 1974), and stimulation of degrading enzymes (Mankin 1982). It is the variability of the repair process that contributes to the difficulty in predicting results of cartilage repair (Buckwalter et al. 1990).

Clinical factors that may influence the maturation and remodeling of the repair tissue include: the location and size (Convery et al. 1972) of the defect; the postoperative management, including continuous passive motion (Salter et al. 1980), the loading history; and the constitution of the patient with respect to age (Buckwalter and Mow 1992), weight, and joint malalignment. The biomechanical properties of reparative tissue may not be sufficient to withstand joint loading, with the subsequent degeneration of the tissue in the defect resulting in a chronic, symptomatic defect of the joint surface (Byers et al. 1970). In order to restore joint function, and to prevent further deterioration of the joint, repair tissue should have structure, composition and mechanical properties of articular cartilage (Radin 1990).

Clinical Treatment of Cartilage Defects

Orthopedic surgeons are still challenged in treating symptomatic full-thickness articular cartilage injuries. Treatments involve several techniques to stimulate bleeding from the subchondral bone to promote clot formation and a subsequent healing cascade, or the use of autologous tissue or cultured cells to facilitate cartilage regeneration. The full regeneration of structure and restoration of function of articular cartilage has not yet been achieved by any of the procedures in animal experiments, and the efficacy in human subjects has not yet been established (Buckwalter et al. 1990). Surgical procedures treating chronic cartilage defects include: abrasion arthroplasty (Johnson 1986), subchondral drilling (Pridie 1959; Tippett 1991) microfracturing (Steadman 1992) and spongialization (Ficat et al. 1979). Perichondrial grafting involves either suturing or gluing rib perichondrium to the defect to introduce chondroprogenitor cells from the perichondrial germinative layer to achieve repair of the defect (Amiel et al. 1985; Engkvist and Johansson 1980; Homminga et al. 1989; Skoog and Johansson 1976). In a recently developed technique, a suspension of cultured autologous chondrocytes is implanted under a periosteal graft, which is sutured to the defect (Brittberg et al. 1994). This technique provides exogenous chondrocytes as a cell source to facilitate cartilage regeneration (Grande et al. 1989). The use of a cell suspension of ex vivo cultured chondrocytes as a source for cartilage repair opened up a new approach for the treatment of defects of the articular surface in joints. The special requirement in the implantation procedure of producing a leak-proof compartment for the injectable cells by suturing a periosteal graft to the articular cartilage defect has prompted continuing efforts to develop biomaterials to serve as cell delivery systems.

Tissue Engineering

Tissue engineering includes the use of cells, matrices and regulators (e.g. growth factors) to synthesize tissues, which by nature do not regenerate or repair sufficiently (Fig. 1). This new-evolving field in a multidisciplinary approach including engineering, biochemistry, molecular biology and medicine to repair defects to restore normal function. In order to engineer articular cartilage in the laboratory, synthetic and natural polymer matrices have been seeded with cells in culture that can adequately replace defective joint surface (Vacanti et al. 1993). Alternatively implants have been produced to facilitate regeneration of articular cartilage in vivo (Green 1977). Cell sources have included: allogeneic or autologous cells isolated from articular cartilage (Bentley and Greer 1971), periosteum (Rich et al. 1994), perichondrium (Chu et al. 1995; Coutts et al. 1994) and mesenchymal

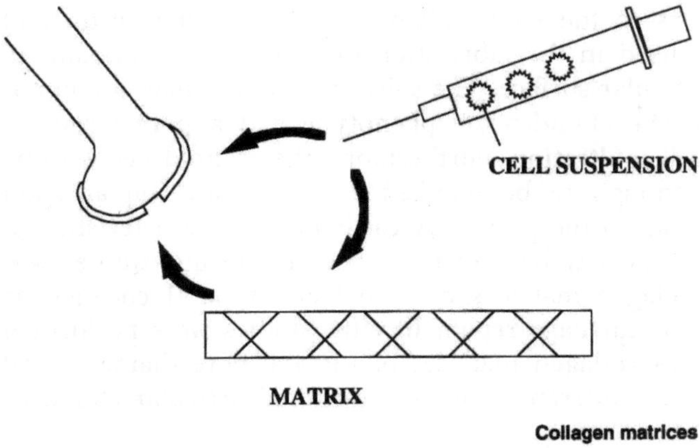

Fig. 1. Approaches in tissue engineering: articular cartilage lesions are treated by implanting cultured cells in cell suspension directly into the defect (e.g. preferably under a periosteal flap) or by using matrices (e.g. collagen matrices) as scaffolds for cell implantation

(stromal) stem cells (Caplan et al. 1993) from bone marrow. In most techniques cells are harvested by enzymatic digestion, expanded in cell culture, and then reimplanted by the use of different scaffolds as vehicles for the cultured cells. In monolayer culture the chondrocytes are able to proliferate but they take on a fibroblast-like phenotype and decrease synthesis of cartilage-specific proteins. In three-dimensional culture conditions the chondrocytes are able to reexpress a chondrocytic phenotype by adopting a spherical morphology in these matrices. It is not yet possible to determine which source of cells will yield the most favorable results. There are advantages and disadvantages for each approach, related to the requirements for harvesting the cells and the potential for regeneration of articular cartilage. In the case of allogeneic cells there is the potential for immune response (Langer and Gross 1974) and infectious complications.

Matrices used as scaffolds for transportation of cultured cells, provide for a uniform cell distribution, and serve to maintain the cells in the target site (Freed et al. 1993). The natural and synthetic polymers employed as scaffolds for engineering articular cartilage include: fibrin (Hendrickson et al. 1993), collagen gels (Kimura et al. 1984) and collagen sponges (Speer et al. 1979) and polyglycolic and polylactic acid (Freed et al. 1994). Gels produced from type I collagen have been used to culture chondrocytes in vitro and to facilitate articular cartilage regeneration in vivo. Insoluble type I collagen matrices have been successful in animal models to improve healing of cartilage defects (Grande et al. 1993). However, complete regeneration was not achieved; the reparative tissue consisted of fibrous and fibrocartilaginous substances with some hyaline cartilage also found.

Questions remain as to the most suitable chemical composition and pore structure to be used in the fabrication of a cell-seeded implant to treat defects in the articular surface. The substance should have a composition that maintains the chondrocyte phenotype and a pore structure that accommodates cell infiltration. Furthermore, the scaffold needs to be mechanically stable enough to be handled surgically for implantation (Nixon et al. 1993). Due to the poor surgical handling characteristics of gels, sponge-like matrices may be preferred. The goal of our studies was to evaluate porous collagen matrices of type I and type II collagen as cell-seeded implants for cartilage repair. In vitro studies were performed using different types of collagen matrices of varying pore diameter and collagen type, as well as different sources of cultured articular chondrocytes.

Collagen Matrices

In Vitro Experiment

In vitro studies were performed to determine attachment and distribution of the seeded cells and the reexpression of the chondrocytic phenotype in type I and type II collagen matrices and to compare the biosynthetic activity of the seeded chondrocytes (Nehrer et al. 1998; Nehrer et al. 1997).

The type I collagen-glycosaminoglycan (GAG) co-polymer was produced as a co-precipitate of type I collagen from bovine hide (Integra Life Science, Plainsboro, N.J., USA) and of chondroitin-6-sulfate from shark cartilage, converted into a highly porous sheet by freeze drying. The matrix was produced with pore diameters of 25 and 85 µm. The type II material produced by treating porcine cartilage (Geistlich Biomaterials, Wolhusen, Switzerland) had a pore size of 85 µm. The type II sponges were cross-linked by ultraviolet-irradiation to decrease the degradation rate and increase mechanical stability (Weadock et al. 1995). Chondrocytes were isolated enzymatically from harvested articular cartilage of the knee joints (patella, tibia) of calves, adult mongrel dogs, and adult human subjects. The cells were cultured in monolayer and passaged one time. After expansion in monolayer the chondrocytes were trypsinized and the cell suspension, containing about one million chondrocytes, was seeded onto the collagen sponges.

At the termination of the experiment after 3 h to 21 days, the specimens were evaluated histologically for cell morphology and cell distribution. Microtomed sections of plastic-embedded specimens were stained with hematoxylin and eosin (HE) and safranin-O. Percentages of cells displaying spherical, chondrocytic morphology and elongated, fibroblastic shape were determined using a grid eyepiece. For assay of cell proliferation and biosynthetic activity the sponges with canine chondrocytes were digested in papain: DNA content was determined using the Hoechst dye number 33258; and the amount of GAG was assessed by measuring the content of chondroitin-4-sulfate by the dimethyl methylene blue method.

Histological analysis of the cell-seeded constructs revealed higher percentages of cells assuming a chondrocytic phenotype (spherical shape) in the type II matrix compared to the type I matrix with comparable pore diameter (85 µm) at all time points and for different species (Fig. 2 a, b).

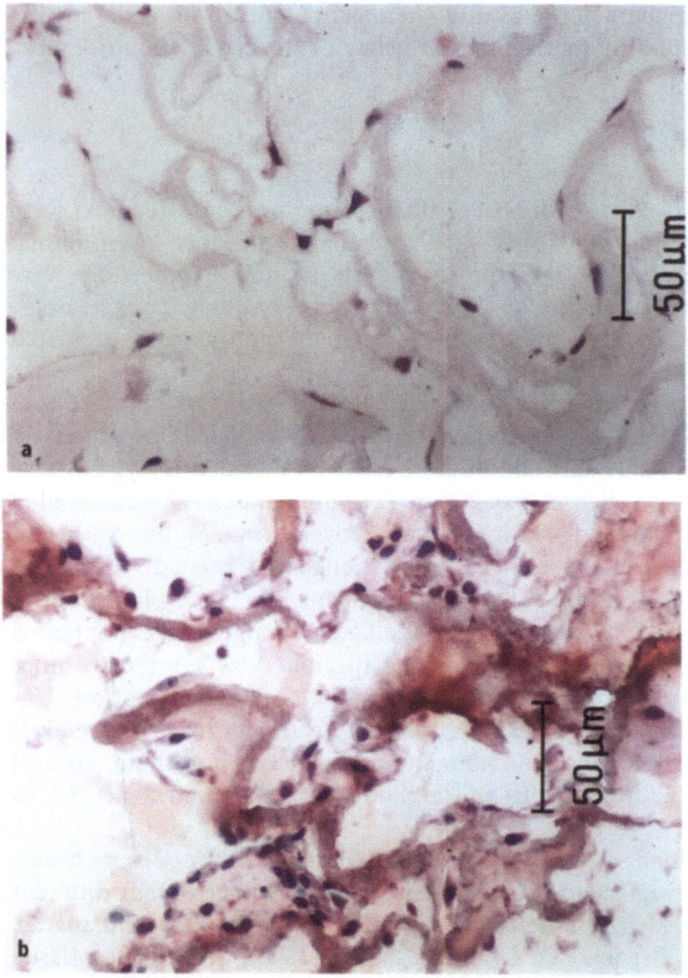

Fig. 2 a, b. Cultured chondrocytes in type I collagen matrices (**a**) assume a fibroblast-like, elongated cell shape, whereas in a type II collagen matrix (**b**) the majority of the cells yielded the chondrocytic, round phenotype (hematoxylin and eosin staining)

Canine chondrocytes in the type I collagen matrix with smaller pore diameter (Kimura et al. 1984) displayed a higher percentage of the chondrocytic phenotype at the early time points (3 h), but no difference after 7 days, compared to the type II matrix (Nehrer et al. 1997). The bioassays revealed significant increases in GAG and DNA over the 7 days of culture. However, the increase of GAG normalized to DNA (μg GAG/μg DNA) was significantly higher in the type II sponge.

The in vitro studies showed that collagen type and pore size influenced the morphology and biosynthetic activity of seeded chondrocytes. The type II collagen matrix yielded the highest percentage of cells with spherical shape and biosynthetic activity at each time period. Our results suggest that the pore characteristics and chemical composition of the matrix are important factors in controlling the behavior of seeded chondrocytes.

In Vivo Experiment

Type I and type II collagen matrices of the same pore size (85 μm) were used as cell-seeded scaffolds in a cartilage repair procedure in an animal model (Nehrer et al. 1998). Chondral defects (4 mm in diameter) were produced in the trochlear groove of the knee joint of adult mongrel dogs. The defects were divided among five treatment groups and evaluated after 16 weeks.

Small pieces of cartilage were harvested from non-articulating areas of the knee joint. Chondrocytes were enzymatically isolated, expanded in cell culture for 12 days, and one million cells were seeded in type II collagen sponges with a diameter of 5 mm (2–3 mm thick). The cell-seeded constructs were implanted within 12 h and covered by a sutured layer of the type II material. The type I collagen sponge was seeded with chondrocytes as described above. The cell-seeded matrices were placed under a sutured fascia flap. Unseeded type I collagen sponges were implanted under the fascia flap and the free fascia flap alone was sutured to other defects as a control to evaluate the influence of cell augmentation. Untreated defects were prepared as controls. All treatment groups were evaluated after 15 weeks. Defects obtained immediately after their surgical preparation and within 30 min of implantation of a matrix served as acute controls.

Paraffin-embedded sections stained with HE and safranin-O were evaluated using a grid eyepiece to determine the area percentage of four different specific tissue types in the defect based on cell morphology and matrix structure: fibrous tissue (FT); hyaline cartilage (HC); "transition" tissue (TT), between FT and HC, including fibrocartilage; and articular cartilage (AC). Bonding of the repair tissue to the subchondral plate and adjacent cartilage, and degradation of the adjacent tissues were documented.

The acute controls revealed only small amounts of remnants of AC and only occasional damage to the subchondral plate. The acute implant controls revealed that the implant was still in place 30 min after joint closure (Fig. 3). Gross appearance after 15 weeks showed the best result for the cell-seeded type II matrix with whitish repair tissue filling the defect; the borders of the defect, however, were clearly visible. Histologically the cell-seeded type II collagen implant group contained the most reparative tissue (i.e. the greatest amount of fill, 58%). The areal percentage of hyaline and articular cartilage was comparable for both types of cell-seeded collagen implants. The subchondral bone displayed a remarkable remodeling process. The unseeded implants and the fascia group contained no hyaline cartilage. The untreated controls displayed less filling, but the highest areal percent of hyaline and articular cartilage. Evaluation of the adjacent cartilage revealed no difference among treatment groups; although remarkable suture damage was found in some sections.

The animal model revealed that cell-seeded implants of both types of collagen of the same pore diameter were able to increase the amount of tissue filling the defect. However, histological analysis of tissue types revealed mostly FT and TT for both types of matrices. In contrast to other animal studies, we did not find an increased formation of hyaline cartilage after implantation of cell seeded constructs in a chondral defect in adult canines at 15 weeks. However, about 80% of the repair tissue after implantation of a seeded type II collagen implant was transition tissue suggesting a maturation process of the tissue. We found less repair tissue and no regeneration of hyaline tissue after implantation of unseeded col-

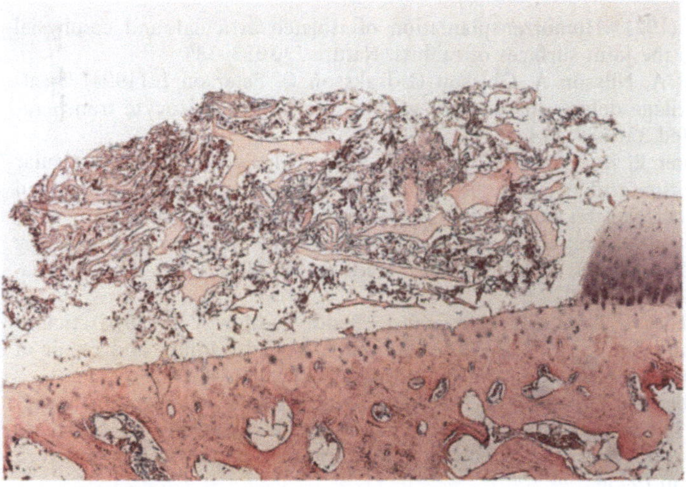

Fig. 3. Histology of a freshly implanted collagen matrix in an experimental defect in a canine model (hematoxylin and eosin staining)

lagen matrices or fascia alone. The areal percentage of hyaline tissue in the untreated defects exceeded that of all of the treatment groups.

Conclusion

Our results demonstrated that cultured chondrocytes seeded in type I and type II collagen matrices proliferate and synthesize cartilage-specific molecules in vitro and can be used as scaffolds for implantation in a chondral defect. Pore characteristics and biochemical composition influenced cell behavior. Although the cell-seeded constructs clearly failed to restore the structure of articular cartilage in the investigated time period, we found an increased tissue formation, which filled the whole defect in many of the specimens. However, some defects showed less filling and the repair process remained unpredictable. Future studies need to investigate long-term follow-up of the increased formation of repair tissue and the subchondral remodeling process. Variation of pore characteristics and chemical composition of matrices, as well as cell sources, culture conditions and seeding techniques have to be investigated to improve regeneration of hyaline tissue by cell-seeded implants.

References

Amiel D, Coutts R, Abel M, Stewart W, Harwood F, Akeson W (1985) Rib perichondrial grafts for the repair of full thickness articular cartilage defects. J Bone Joint Surg 67A:911–920

Bentley G, Greer R (1971) Homotransplantation of isolated articular and epiphysial chondrocytes into the joint surfaces of rabbits. Nature 230:383–385

Brittberg M, Lindahl A, Nilsson A, Ohlsson C, Isaksson O, Peterson L (1994) Treatment of deep cartilage defects in the knee with autologous chondrocyte transplantation. N Eng J Med 331:889–894

Buckwalter J, Hunziker E, Rosenberg L, Coutts R, Adams M, Eyre D (1988) Articular cartilage: composition and structure. In: Woo SL-J, Buckwalter JA (eds) Injury and repair of the musculoskeletal soft tissues. AAOS, Park Ridge, IL, pp 405–425

Buckwalter J, Mow V (1992) in: Osteoarthritis: Diagnosis and Management, edited by Moskowitz RW, Howell DS, Goldberg VM, Mankin HJ (2nd Edit) Philadelphia, WB Saunders, 1992, pp 71–107

Buckwalter J, Rosenberg L, Coutts R, Hunzider E, Reddi A, Mow V (1988) Articular cartilage: injury and repair. In: Woo SL-J, Buckwalter JA (eds) Injury and repair of the musculoskeletal soft tissues. AAOS, Park Ridge, IL, pp 465–482

Buckwalter J, Rosenberg L, Hunziker E (1990) Articular cartilage composition, structure, response to injury, and methods of facilitating repair. In: Ewing JW (eds) Articular cartilage and knee joint function: basic science and arthroscopy. Raven Press, New York, pp 19–56

Byers P, Conteponti C, Farkas T (1970) A post-mortem study of the hip joint. Ann Rheum Dis 29:15–31

Caplan A, Fink D, Goto T, Linton A, Young R, Wakitani S, Goldberg V, Haynesworth S (1993) Mesenchymal stem cells and tissue repair. Raven Press, New York
Chu C, Coutts D, Yoshioka M, Harwood L, Monosov A, Amiel D (1995) Articular cartilage repair using allogenic perichondrocyte-seeded biodegradable poly-lactic acid (PLA): a tissue engineering study. J Biomed Mat Res 29:1147–1154
Convery FR, Akeson WH, Keown GH (1972) The repair of large osteochondral defects. An experimental study in horses. Clin Orthop Rel Res 82:253–262
Coutts R, Yoshioka M, Amiel D, Hacker S, Harwood F, Monosov A (1994) Cartilage repair using a porous polylactic acid matrix with allogenic perichondrial cells. 40th ORS Meeting, New Orleans, pp 240–241
Engkvist O, Johansson SH (1980) Perichondrial arthroplasty: a clinical study in twenty-six patients. Scand J Plast Reconstr Surg 14:71–87
Ficat R, Ficat C, Gedeon P, Toussaint J (1979) Spongialization: a new treatment for diseased patellae. Clin Orthop 144:74–83
Freed L, Marquis J, Nohria A, Emmanual J, Mikos A, Langer R (1993) Neocartilage formation in vitro and in vivo using cells cultured on synthetic biodegradable polymers. J Biomed Mat Res 27:11–23
Freed LE, Grande DA, Lingbin Z, Emmanual J, Marquis JC, Langer R (1994) Joint resurfacing using allograft chondrocytes and synthetic biodegradable polymer scaffolds. J Biomed Mater Res 28:891–899
Grande DA, Pitman MI, Peterson L, Menche D, Klein M (1989) The repair of experimentally produced defects in rabbit articular cartilage by autologous chondrocyte transplantation. J Orthop Res 7:208–218
Grande D, Halberstadt C, Schwartz R, Linton J, Naughton G (1993) Evaluation of extracellular matrix scaffolds for engineering of articular cartilage grafts. 39th ORS Meeting, San Francisco, p 227
Green W (1977) Articular cartilage repair. Behavior of rabbit chondrocytes during tissue culture and subsequent allografting. Clin Orthop Rel Res 124:327–250
Hendrickson D, Nixon A, Erb H, Lust G (1993) Phenotype and biological activity of neonatal equine chondrocytes cultured in a three-dimensional fibrin matrix. Am J Vet Res 55:410–414
Homminga G, van der Linden T, Terwindt-Rouwenhorst E, Drukker J (1989) Repair of articular defects by perichondrial grafts: experiments in the rabbit. Acta Orthop Scand 60:326–329
Hunter W (1743) On the structure and disease of articulating cartilage. Philos Trans R Soc Lond B Biol Sci 42b:514–521
Johnson L (1991) Characteristics of the immediate postarthroscopic blood clot formation in the knee joint. Arthroscopy 7:14–23
Johnson LL (1986) Arthroscopic abrasion arthroplasty historical and pathologic perspective: present status. Arthroscopy 2:54–69
Kimura T, Yasui N, Ohsawa S, Ono K (1984) Chondrocytes embedded in collagen gels maintain cartilage phenotype during long-term cultures. Clin Orthop Rel Res 186: 231–239
Langer F, Gross A. (1974) Immunogenicity of allograft articular cartilage. J Bone Joint Surg 56A:297–304
Mankin H, Mow V, Buckwalter J, Iannotti J, Ratcliffe A (1994) Form and function of articular cartilage. In: Sheldon R Simon (ed) American Academy of Orthopedic Surgeons. Orthopedic Basic Science, pp 1–44
Mankin HJ (1982) The response of articular cartilage to mechanical injury. J Bone Joint Surg 64A:460–466
Nehrer S, Breinan H, Ashkar S, Shortkroff S, Minas T, Sledge C, Yannas J, Spector M (1998) Characteristics of articular chondrocytes seeded in collagen matrices in vitro. Tissue Engineering 4:175–183

Nehrer S, Breinan H, Ramappa A, Hsu H-P, Shortkroff S, Minas T, Spector M (1998) Autologous chondrocyte-seeded type I and type II collagen matrices implanted in a chondral defect in a canine model. ORS, New Orleans, p 377

Nehrer S, Breinan H, Ramappa A, Shortkroff S, Young G, Minas T, Sledge C, Yannas J, Spector M (1998) Canine chondrocytes seeded in type I and type II collagen implants investigated in vitro. J Biomed Mat Res 38:95–104

Nehrer S, Breinan H, Ramappa A, Young G, Shortkroff S, Louie L, Sledge C, Yannas J, Spector M (1997) Matrix collagen type and pore size influence behavior of seeded canine chondrocytes. Biomaterials 18:769–776

Nixon A, Sams A, Lust G, Grande D, Mohammed H (1993) Temporal matrix synthesis and histological features of a chondrocyte laden porous collagen analogue. Am J Vet Res 54:349–356

Paget J (1853) Healing of injuries in various tissues. Lect Surg Pathol T:262

Pridie K (1959) A method of resurfacing osteoarthritic knee joints. J Bone Joint Surg 41B:618–619

Radin E (1990) Factors influencing osteoarthrosis progression. Raven Press, New York

Rich D, Johnson E, Zhou L, Grande D (1994) The use of periosteal cell/polymer tissue constructs for the repair of articular cartilage defects. 40th ORS meeting, New Orleans, p 241

Rodrigo JJ, Steadman RJ, Siliman JF, Fulstone HA (1994) Improvement of fullthickness chondral defects in the human knee after debridement and microfracture using continous passive motion. Am J Knee Surg 7(3):109–116

Salter RB, Simmonds DF, Malcolm BW, Rumble EJ, MacMichael D (1980) The biological effect of continuous passive motion on the healing of full-thickness defects in articular cartilage. J Bone Joint Surg 62A:1232–1251

Skoog T, Johansson SH (1976) The formation of articular cartilage from free perichondrial grafts. Plast Reconstr Surg 57:1–6

Speer D, Chvapil M, Volz R, Holmes M (1979) Enhancement of healing in osteochondral defects by collagen implantation. Clin Orthop Rel Res 144:326–335

Tippett J (1991) Articular cartilage drilling and osteotomy. In: JB McGinty et al. (eds) Osteoarthritis of the knee. Operative arthroscopy. Raven Press, New York, pp 325–339

Vacanti C, Kim W, Upton J, Schloo G, Vacanti J (1993) Tissue engineered composites of bone and cartilage using synthetic polymers seeded with two cell types. 39th ORS meeting, San Francisco, p 276

Weadock K, Miller E, Bellincampi L, Zawadsky J (1995) Physical crosslinking of collagen fibers: comparison of ultraviolet irradiation and dehydrothermal treatment. J Biomed Mat Res 29:1373–1379

Autologous Chondrocyte Grafting for the Treatment of Cartilage Defects

M. Brittberg

Introduction

The repair of a damaged tissue is typically dependent on the formation of a blood clot. This blood clot eventually fills the damaged tissue area and attracts cells from the surrounding tissue that can repair the injured area. The resultant scar tissue in time matures to become almost identical to the original tissue.

Adult articular cartilage lacks blood vessels and when the cartilage is damaged, a blood clot does not form. The defect area will not heal (Buckwalter and Cruess 1991). A small defect may not cause any trouble but larger defects will give rise to locking or catching of the knee, local pain and swelling. Some of these defects may also progress to the more widespread joint failure of osteoarthritis. There are a substantial number of patients suffering from disabling joint complaints due to different degrees of cartilage damage. The methods used to treat this joint damage have so far not been very successful (Buckwalter and Lohmander 1994).

Formation of cartilage during both embryonic development and repair processes involves the differentiation of so-called multipotential primitive mesenchymal cells. These cells exist, for example, in muscle, bone-marrow, periosteum and rib cartilage. In a milieu without blood vessels, they can start to produce a cartilaginous tissue.

Principles of Repair Mechanisms

In the injured site, a cell-dependent-differentiation occurs. This means that the initial number of cells that are able to take part in the repair events is of great importance. In the defect area, primitive mesenchymal stem cells undergo a series of cellular transitions with an ultimate differentiation to the original phenotype of the injured tissue. This repair lineage is common to all types of mesenchymal tissue (Caplan 1991; Caplan et al. 1993). The repair of the mesenchymal tissue is thus dependent on the local availability of these stem cells. The goal for the surgeon is to supply high densities of these repair-competent cells to the injured site, such as a chondral defect, to achieve some sort of repair or healing.

Each type of repair of chondral defects can be seen as the introduction of cells into the injury area. Investigators all over the world have tried to use these primitive cells to repair cartilage defects by drilling the lesions to attract bone marrow cells (Buckwalter and Lohmander 1994; Pridie 1959), resurfacing with periosteum (Angermann and Riegels-Nielsen 1994; Niedermann et al. 1985; O'Driscoll et al. 1986) and perichondrium (Beckers et al. 1992; Engkvist 1979; Homminga et al. 1990). This type of so called "biological resurfacing" has been promising in young animal trials but not sufficiently studied in humans. The cells that could be used and the cells that are able to induce a hyaline repair that will withstand wear are open to discussion. Several techniques for cartilage repair describe the repair as hyaline-like due to the hyaline appearance in morphology and/or biochemistry but no one has achieved cartilage regeneration; a full restoration of the structure identical to the original tissue. All these cell sources may prove effective in the creation of a functional tissue-engineered graft, but those that are best remain to be discussed.

The chondrocytes do not divide to any large extent in animal or human cartilage. But if the cells are separated from the cartilage matrix they can be expanded in vitro. The cells can be cultured for 2–3 weeks to expand the number of cells 20–30 times the initial amount.

Animal Studies

This knowledge was used by Lars Peterson and co-workers in 1982 when they developed a rabbit model to treat cartilage defects in the rabbit patella with their own cultured cells (Grande et al. 1989). With that model, using the knee joints of adult rabbits, Grande and co-workers (1989) examined the effect of autologous chondrocytes grown in vitro on the healing rate of chondral defects not penetrating the subchondral bone plate. To determine whether any of the reconstituted cartilage resulted from the chondrocyte graft an experiment was conducted involving grafts with chondrocytes that had been labeled prior to grafting with a nuclear tracer. Results were evaluated using both qualitative and quantitative light microscopy. Macroscopic results from grafted specimens displayed a marked decrease in synovitis and other degenerative changes. In defects that had received transplants, a significant amount of cartilage was reconstituted (82%) compared to ungrafted controls (18%). Autoradiography on reconstituted cartilage showed that there were labeled cells incorporated into the repair matrix.

The above-mentioned rabbit model has since then been used and further developed by our group in Göteborg. The cultured cells are injected into a pre-made cartilage defect in the patella of the rabbit and covered with a flap of periosteum, functioning as a biological membrane. This method resulted in a high degree of healed rabbit patellar defects and the repair tissue was similar to the original cartilaginous tissue (Brittberg et al. 1996).

In mature articular cartilage, the chondrocyte is a resting cell and functions in a well-regulated, balanced system between the chondrocyte and matrix. An insult or injury, like the enzymatic digestion of matrix, will start cell proliferation and permit the rapid expansion of the number of cells available. The isolated chondrocytes are phenotypically unstable and will dedifferentiate in the monolayer culture system that we use for cell culture. However, the cells regain the chondrocytic phenotype when the cultured cells are encapsulated with their own newly produced matrix (Brittberg 1996; Brittberg et al. 1996). It is possible that the isolation of chondrocytes and the expansion of cells in culture until confluence with most of the cells still dedifferentiated is the ideal way to obtain a large number of mesenchymal cells which, after seeding, continue to produce a hyaline cartilaginous tissue until the cells go into terminal differentiation.

In our rabbit model we never opened the subchondral space in the defects and the defect area was thus an area of low oxygen tension with no contact with the host vasculature (Brittberg 1996; Brittberg et al. 1996). This is also important in order to retain the phenotypic stability of the chondrocytes. After drilling chondral lesions, invading mesenchymal stem cells could differentiate into chondrocytes, but these cells could eventually produce fibrocartilage containing amounts of type I collagen. This might occur under the influence of vascular-derived factors such as a high oxygen tension and specific growth factors. This fact could be of importance when studying the cell repair in different animals bearing in mind the different qualities of the subchondral bone in different species. The subchondral bone in the rabbit patella is quite hard and difficult to break through during the preparation for cell transplantation. The subchondral bone in the pig and dog is much thinner and one could easily go through the bone plate and eventually jeopardize the repair (Breinan et al. 1997).

An opening of the subchondral space could thus negatively influence the repair of a cartilage defect seeded with cultured chondrocytes due to the influence of bioactive vascular factors or ingrowth of other types of mesenchymal cells.

We could regard the cartilage defect as a bioactive chamber (Brittberg 1996). Repair could hypothetically come from the surrounding cartilage in the walls of the defect, from the calcified zone chondrocytes in the cryptae of the irregular subchondral bone plate. Cells could possibly migrate into the defect from the synovial fluid. We know that the cells in the adjacent cartilage show mitotic activity some time after injury but not enough for any significant repair.

Bioactive Chamber

The bioactive chamber theory is useful when alternative cell or tissue transplantation techniques in particular are discussed. Periosteal resurfacing, for instance, is almost always combined with an opening of the subchondral bone marrow space. The periosteal cells and bone marrow cells have dual phenotypic expression and are capable of differentiating to bone and/or cartilage depending on local environmental factors emanating from the vascular bone marrow and from the synovial fluid. However, in contrast to the cartilage nodule formation seen after pure chondrocyte implantation in the athymic mouse, the implantation of periosteally derived cells into the subcutis of an athymic mouse will produce a nodule consisting of a central portion of cartilage that is slowly turned into bone via endochondral ossification, while the periphery develops into bone through intramembranous bone formation (Nakahara et al. 1990). One theory is that the cells follow their initial program of differentiation and that chondrocytes are committed to produce cartilage, while the periosteal and bone-marrow cells are committed to produce bone. This implies that the chondrocytes developed from both these cell types are pre-stage of osteoblasts. Low oxygen tension and chondrogenic factors will help to retain their chondrogenic status in the osteogenic lineage, but they may be more unstable than the purely committed chondrocytes and progress into hypertrophic chondrocytes and finally into bone. The phenotypic fate thus appears to determine the type of the final tissue.

A factor in favor of the use of committed chondrocytes in transplantation is that there is an age-dependent decline in the number of these multipotential chondrocyte progenitor cells in the periosteum, perichondrium and the bone marrow (Caplan et al. 1993; Nakahara et al. 1990). This knowledge is important as it restricts the use of these tissues to young patients.

Role of the Periosteum

In our rabbit work (Brittberg et al. 1996), the patellar defects were treated with autologous chondrocytes together with a covering periosteal graft on one side. The contra-lateral side was treated with periosteum alone. The defects were deep, reaching down to the calcified zone but with no opening of the subchondral space. In a defect of this type without any treatment, there was an intrinsic repair of 29% of the total defect area, primarily by what we call matrix flow from mitotic activity at the edges of the defect. This level of repair should be compared with the mean repair area of 30% 1 year after periosteal grafting alone and significantly different from the 87% repair area with chondrocytes and periosteum. Consequently, it does not appear that the periosteum makes any significant contribution to the repair. In other reports where successful repair with periosteum has been reported, this repair has been combined with an opening of the subchondral space making it possible for repair-competent cells to invade the defect. These findings may all be explained within the previously mentioned concept of a bioactive chamber as a prerequisite for any cartilage repair.

We have also studied the interaction between the periosteum and the cultured chondrocytes and found that the periosteum stimulated the chondrocytes to proliferate by exerting a paracrine effect on the chondrocyte cloning efficiency (Brittberg 1996). Another important finding was that there were different degrees of differentiation in the chondrocytes in the cultures that responded differently to the periosteal stimulation. The bioactive chamber concept could be used to explain results without cell seeding but with an opening of the subchondral space. In these cases, we can postulate that the periosteum exerts the same paracrine effect on invading mesenchymal stem cells from the bone marrow as it does on transplanted chondrocytes. In young individuals, osteochondrogenic cells from the periosteal cambium layer could directly also contribute to the repair but perhaps even these cells require information from another cell type.

Clinical Use

These animal studies encouraged our group in Göteborg to start to use the technique with human patients in 1987. With the permission from the Swedish ethics committee we started to treat patients with chronic disabling symptoms of the knee joint with cultured cartilage cells from their own cartilage (Fig. 1). The first 23 patients (mean age 27 years) were presented in 1994 (Brittberg et al. 1994a). Those patients had local deep cartilage injuries that had been treated with conventional methods without any healing. The technique appeared to be most successful in patients who had injuries on the femoral surfaces producing a single, localized deep cartilage lesion compared with the patella patients that were less successful. This morphology is important to note, as opposed to the gradual wear and tear of advancing age and arthritis. The disappointing outcome of the patella group might have resulted from mechanical misalignments of the patella that were not corrected at the time of transplant surgery.

A new examination was done in 1996 on 92 patients with a follow-up between 2–9 years. There was a high percentage of good to excellent results in patients with single femoral condyle lesions (24 patients, 92%)

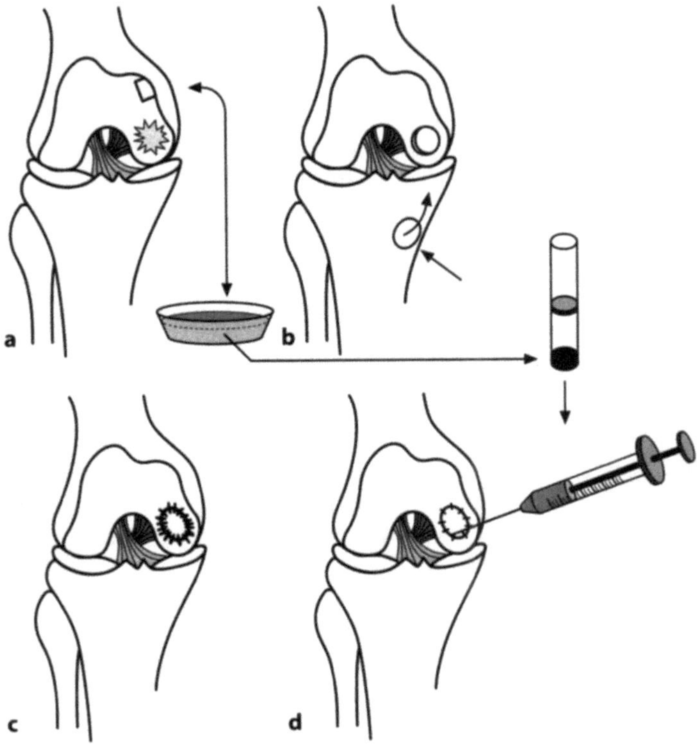

Fig. 1 a–d. a A cartilage injury on the medial femoral condyle has been found. Cartilage slices (300–500 mg) are harvested from an unloaded area on the upper medial femoral condyle. The harvested cartilage is taken to the laboratory and the chondrocytes are isolated and cultured in a nutritional medium for 2 weeks. **b** Two weeks after initial arthroscopy, the joint is opened and the cartilage injury is carefully debrided. A flap of periosteum is taken from the medial tibia to function as a biological membrane. **c** The periosteal flap is sutured over the defect with interrupted resorbable sutures. A fibrin-glue is used to seal the suture row. **d** The cultured cells (8–12 million chondrocytes) in a syringe (0.2–0.4 ml) are injected into the defect below the periosteal flap

and in patients with osteochondritis dissecans (19 patients, 89%) whereas 75% good to excellent results in patients with femoral condyle lesions and a concomitant anterior cruciate injury and ligament reconstruction (16 patients). Twenty-one patella grafted patients were improved in 62% and 75% improved in multiple lesions patients (12 patients). Twenty-six knees were biopsied and 80% of the biopsies showed a hyaline-like appearance.

By January 1998 our cartilage-group in Göteborg had treated 550 patients with disabling cartilage injuries with their own cultured cartilage cells.

Conclusion

Cartilage defect repair requires a continually evolving network of interactions among the implanted cells, surrounding tissue and the produced cytokines. The ongoing basic research is now focused on cytokines and different integrins that can be used to assist in biomaterial-guided tissue regeneration (Brittberg et al. 1994a; Brittberg et al. 1996). Novel polymers are being created and assembled into three-dimensional configurations, to which cells attach and grow to reconstitute tissues. However, it is a difficult task to find a scaffold that is resorbed at the same speed as the neocartilage is formed.

Focal cartilage destruction is the major feature of the disease of osteoarthritis afflicting about 75% of the elderly population. To what extent a single lesion of the cartilage will progress into osteoarthritis is not known. It is possible to use different methods to repair a destroyed articular surface to a greater or lesser degree but we do not know the natural course of a chondral injury. Which lesion will progress and which will not? It is also not known if repairing a local cartilage defect with a good quality repair cartilage will prevent such a development.

The future of cartilage injury treatment may possibly be found in a bioengineering approach, programming cells or tissues to repair the chondral and osteochondral injuries.

References

Angermann P, Riegels-Nielsen P (1994) Osteochondritis dissecans of the femoral condyle treated with periosteal transplantation. A preliminary clinical study of 14 patients. Orthopaedics 2:425–428

Beckers JMH, Bulstra SK, Kuijer R, Bouwmeester SJM, van der Linden AJ (1992) Analysis of the clinical results after perichondral transplantation for cartilage defects of the human knee (abstract). 19th symposium of the ESOA-Joint Destruction and Osteoarthritis, Nordwijkerhout, Netherlands, p 157

Breinan HA, Minas T, Hsu H-P, Nehrer S, Sledge CB, Spector M (1997) Effect of cultured autologous chondrocytes on repair of chondral defects in a canine model. J Bone Joint Surg 79A:1439–1451

Brittberg M, Faxèn E, Peterson L (1994a) Carbon fiber scaffolds in the treatment of early knee osteoarthritis. A prospective 4-year follow-up of 37 patients. Clin Orthop 307:155–164

Brittberg M, Lindahl A, Nilsson A, Ohlsson C, Isaksson O, Peterson L (1994b) Treatment of deep cartilage defects in the knee with autologous chondrocyte transplantation. N Engl J Med 331:889–895

Brittberg M (1996) Cartilage repair. On cartilaginous tissue engineering with the emphasis on autologous chondrocyte transplantation (Thesis). University of Göteborg, Göteborg

Brittberg M, Nilsson A, Lindahl A, Ohlsson C, Peterson L (1996) Rabbit articular cartilage defects in the knee with autologous cultured chondrocytes. Clin Orthop Rel Res 326:270–283

Buckwalter JA, Cruess R (1991) Healing of musculoskeletal tissues. In: Rockwood CA, Green DP, Bucholtz RW (eds) Fractures in adults, 3rd edn, Lippincott, Philadelphia, pp 181–222

Buckwalter JA, Lohmander S (1994) Operative treatment of osteoarthritis: current practice and future development. J Bone Joint Surg 76A:1405–1418

Caplan AI (1991) Mesenchymal stem cells. J Orthop Res 9:641–650

Caplan AI, Fink DJ, GotoT, Linton AE, Young RG, Wakitani S, Goldberg VM, Haynesworth SE (1993) Mesenchymal stem cells and tissue repair. In: Jackson DW Arnoczky SP, Frank CB, Woo SL-Y, Simon TM (eds) The anterior cruciate ligament: current and future concepts. Raven Press, New York, pp 405–417

Engkvist O (1979) Reconstruction of patellar articular cartilage with free autologous perichondrial grafts. Scand J Plast Reconstr Surg 13:361–369

Grande DA, Pitman MI, Peterson L, Menche D, Klein M (1989) The repair of experimentally produced defects in rabbit articular cartilage by autologous chondrocyte transplantation. J Orthop Res 7:208–218

Homminga G, Bulstra SK, Bouwmeester PSM, van der Linden AJ (1990) Perichondral grafting for cartilage lesions of the knee. J Bone Joint Surg 72B:1003–1007

Nakahara H, Bruder SP, Goldberg VM, Caplan AI (1990) On vivo osteochondrogenic potential of cultured cells derived from the periosteum. Clin Orthop 259:223–232

Niedermann B, Boe SD, Lauritzen J, Rubak JM (1985) Glued periosteal grafts in the knee. Acta Orthop Scand 56:457–460

O'Driscoll SW, Keeley FW, Salter RB (1986) The chondrogenic potential of free autogenous periosteal grafts for biological resurfacing of major full thickness defects in joint surfaces under the influence of continuous passive motion. J Bone Joint Surg 68A:1017–1035

Peterson L (1997) Treatment of articular cartilage lesions and osteochondritis dissicans with autologous cultured chondrocytes in the human knee. 2nd Fribourg International Symposium on Cartilage repair. Fribourg, Switzerland 59, Abstract

Pridie KH (1959) A method of resurfacing osteoarthritic knee joints. J Bone Joint Surg 41B:618–619

Perichondrial Grafting for the Treatment of Hyalin Cartilage Defects – Experimental In Vitro and In Vivo Data

J. Bruns

Introduction

The effectiveness of autologous rib perichondrium for repair of full-thickness hyaline cartilage defects has been shown experimentally and clinically in various reports (Amiel et al. 1985a, 1985b, 1988; Bruns et al. 1992, 1994; Bulstra et al. 1990; Coutts et al. 1984). The purpose of these two studies was to examine the behavior of sheep rib perichondrial tissue under in vitro conditions depending on different culture conditions; and in vivo depending on the anatomical side and fixation technique in a large animal model (Bruns et al. 1992, 1994).

In Vitro Examination

Materials and Methods

Rib perichondrium was obtained from sheep used for an experimental in vivo trial. Specimens were cultured for 14 days under standard culture conditions. The explants were initially cultured on collagen sponges (group A), fibrin glue (group B) and cellulose acetate filter (group C). Then, in the second part with or without the addition of fetal calf serum (FCS). Specimens were examined histologically, histochemically, histomorphometrically and autoradiographically (Bruns et al. 1994).

Results

Histologically, a clear differentiation of perichondrial cells towards a chondrocyte-like cell shape particularly in the proliferation zone was noticed on all three matrices. These cells synthesized new matrix substances comparable to the ground substance normally present in hyaline cartilage (Fig. 4 and 5).

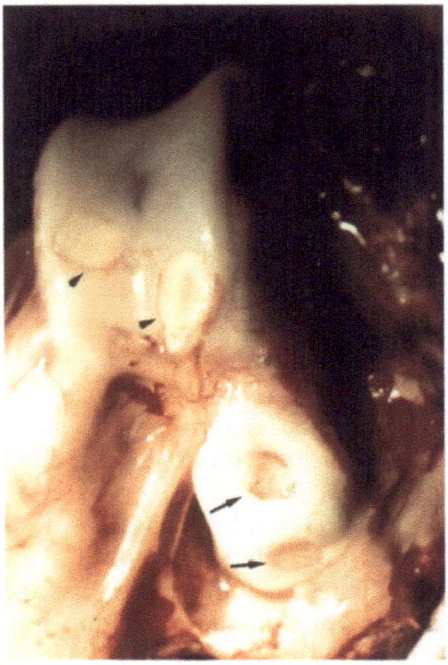

Fig. 1. Sheep knee joint with two drill-holes, 7 mm in diameter, in the non-weight-bearing area (patellar groove, *arrowheads*) and two drill-holes in the weight-bearing area at the femoral condyle (*arrows*) filled with perichondrial grafts: after 8 weeks a complete filling in the non-weight-bearing areas and incomplete filling in the weight-bearing area is visible

Autoradiographic analysis using 3-*H*-thymidine demonstrated the proliferation zone as the most proliferative area. Morphometric analyses of the tissue differentiation due to the use of different culture matrices revealed no significant differences in the proliferation rates (Bruns et al. 1994) but a significant increase with time (Fig. 6).

A clear differentiation of perichondrial cells towards a chondrocyte-like cell shape was also noticed when FCS was not added (Fig. 6).

In Vivo Examination

Materials and Methods

Osteochondral lesions were made in the articular surface of knee joints in 36 sheep. The defects were filled with autologous rib perichondrial grafts that were secured by either collagen sponges ($n=12$ animals) or fibrin glue ($n=12$ animals). Defects without perichondrial grafts served as controls ($n=12$ animals). Following 1 week of immobilization of the operated leg, the plaster was removed and the animals were allowed to move freely. Animals were killed after 4, 8, 12 and 16 weeks. The grafts were removed and investigated morphologically (Bruns et al. 1992).

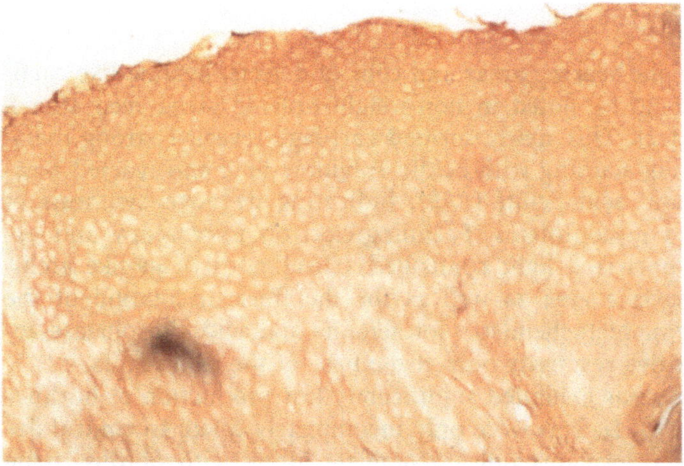

Fig. 2. Microscopic findings in a graft 8 weeks after transplantation harvested from the non-weight-bearing area: the superficial zone (*top*) exhibits newly produced cartilage with a high density of chondrons (v. Gieson ×16)

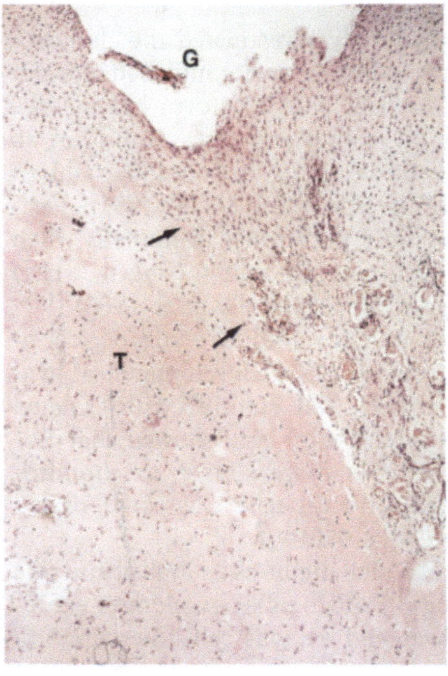

Fig. 3. Microscopic finding in a graft 4 weeks after transplantation into a weight-bearing area: area between graft (*T*) and normal cartilage: Surface (*G*) is depressed and the rim towards the normal cartilage (*arrows*) is filled with scar tissue containing blood vessels (hematoxylin and eosin [HE]×96)

Results

In contrast to weight-bearing areas and control defects, hyaline-like cartilage formation could be noted in non-weight-bearing areas even after 4 weeks (Fig. 1 and 2). This newly formed cartilage revealed strong metachromasia following staining with acidic Toluidine-blue and reacted positively with periodic acid–Schiff (PAS), indicating de novo synthesis of proteoglycans and glycoproteins. Scanning-electron microscopy and examinations with polarized light confirmed a hyaline-cartilage-like architecture for the surface area as well as for the fiber orientation of the whole graft. Enzyme histochemistry for alkaline and acid phosphatase activity showed positive reactivity only at the base of the transplants.

Weight-bearing areas exhibited significantly less production of hyaline-like cartilage (Fig. 3). Defects were only incompletely filled. In control defects without any transplants only incomplete filling with fibrous tissue was seen (Bruns et al. 1992).

Discussion

Tizzoni (1878) and Doerner (1905) had already investigated the chondrogenic potential of perichondrium. Other authors have confirmed the potential of this specific tissue as perichondrial grafts to form hyaline-like cartilage in articular cartilage lesions in rabbits and dogs (Amiel et al. 1985; Engkvist and Ohlsen 1979; Engkvist et al. 1979; Kon 1981; Ohlsen and Widenfalk (1983); Skoog et al. 1972, 1975; Woo et al. 1987). Perichondrial grafting has also been successfully performed in humans when the grafts were applied into non-weight-bearing joints (finger, wrist) (Pastacaldi and Engkvist 1979; Serradge et al. 1984; Sully et al. 1980).

In contrast, only a small number of in vitro studies using perichondrial tissue have been performed (Bruns et al. 1994). Development of hyaline-like cartilage was clearly demonstrated. Cell cultures with isolated perichondrial cells (Upton et al. 1981) from rabbit ears showed that isolated perichondrocytes display characteristics more similar to chondrocytes than to fibroblasts. Recently, the in vitro capacity was corroborated for human rib perichondrium (Bulstra et al. 1990).

The rationale for the use of these particular methods is that fibrin glue is commonly used for in vivo graft fixation. Also collagen sponges exhibit a stimulating effect on the cartilaginous and osseous cell differentiation as known from several in vitro investigations (Kimura et al. 1984; Maor et al. 1987; Wakitani et al. 1989; Yasui et al. 1982).

Our results confirm the typical course of cell differentiation towards a hyaline-like cell differentiation. In contrast to Bulstra et al. (1990), we suggest the proliferation zone of the perichondrium to be the most active area for this production. This is based on the observation that cells of the proliferation zone, called perichondrocytes, exhibit the most impressive configural changes from an elongated cell configuration towards a more chondrocytic configuration. This is confirmed by the accompanying histochemical reaction and autoradiographic activity and the fact that perichondrocytes from the proliferation zone demonstrate a chondrocytic configuration as in the transition zone after some days in culture.

A suggested constant promoting effect on cartilaginous cell differentiation due to the use of collagen sponges could not be observed. Neither was there any evidence of deteriorating effects as suggested by Itay et al. (1987), nor signs of stimulating influences on the development of hyaline-like cartilage were detectable by using xenologous fibrin glue as a culture matrix. Comparison of results from grafts cultured on collagen sponges and fibrin glue demonstrated no constant significant differences in the proliferating capacity of perichondrium. From these in vitro data no preference for the use of either fibrin glue or collagen sponge as a gluing agent can be given. Furthermore, we found that even without addition of FCS, perichondrial tissue culture is possible. This opens the opportunity to further examine the influence of growth factors.

For a clinical in vivo application in weight-bearing joints such as knee, ankle and hip, several questions arise regarding the fixation of the grafts, the time of immobilization as well as the mode of mobilization. That is to say that we had to evaluate the role of continuous passive motion (CPM) or active motion (Amiel et al. 1985a, 1985b; Engkvist and Ohlsen 1979; Kon 1981; Salter et al. 1975, 1980). It was therefore the purpose of our in vivo experiment to examine the influence of weight-bearing or weight-restriction on the differentiation of perichondrial grafts into hyaline-like cartilage in a large animal model.

In order to simulate restriction from weight-bearing, perichondrium transplantation was performed at the patellar groove, which has been reported to never come into contact with another joint surface (Passl et al. 1976). These grafts were compared with those transplanted into the weight-bearing area at the femoral condyle that is always in contact with the tibial plateau. Radiographically, it was confirmed that the area defined as "non-weight bearing" had no contact with any other part of the joint in flexion and extension. It was also verified that the area defined as "weight-bearing" was in contact with the tibial plateau.

The sheep were allowed to move freely with active motion. This meant that the two different articular cartilage areas represent two different conditions of active motion with and without weight-bearing. Irrespective of whether the exact conditions of weight-bearing were completely definable, this study clearly demonstrated the different extent of development of a hyaline-like cartilage dependent on the weight-bearing conditions provided in this sheep model. From structural aspects, all micromorphological methods used in this study showed histological and histochemical differentiation from original perichondrial tissue into hyaline-like cartilage up to 16 weeks postoperatively. The development of hyaline-like cartilage followed a typical course. At 4 and 8 weeks after transplantation, remnants of the original fibrous perichondrial part were still visible. After 12 weeks cells of the grafts began to orientate more perpendicular in the deeper part and horizontally in the superficial layer.

Parallel to that, grafts demonstrated an orientation of the fibers similar to the original perichondrial tissue after 4 and 8 weeks, increasing after 12 weeks and even more after 16 weeks (Fig. 2). Fibers began to become orientated more like in normal hyaline cartilage with the typical structure of the superficial, intermediate and deep layer.

The second purpose of the in vivo study was to examine different fixation techniques. Fibrin glue is known to be a sufficiently resorbable glue that is used clinically for refixation of osteochondral fractures and transplants (Coutts et al. 1984; Gaudernak et al. 1986; Homminga et al. 1989, 1990; Kaplonyi et al. 1988; Keller et al. 1986; Passl et al. 1976). Collagen sponges have a good hemostatic function (Schittek et al. 1976). Previous in vitro studies suggest that collagen sponges can promote differentiation of isolated cartilage precursor cells into cartilage and bone cells (Kimura et al. 1984; Maor et al. 1987; Wakitani et al. 1989; Yasui et al. 1982). In our experiment, there were no cartilage differentiation promoting effects.

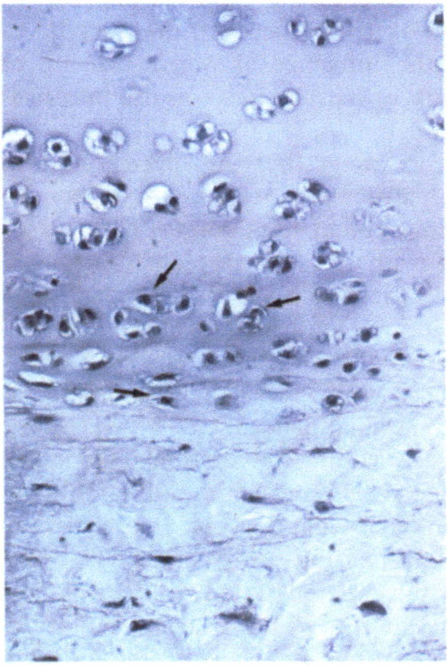

Fig. 4. Perichondrial tissue after 14 days in culture (area between fibrous perichondrium and proliferation zone). The proliferation zone (*arrows*) exhibits some perichondrocytes with a fibrocytic shape, mostly cells with a chondrocytic shape, lying in chondrons, are visible. In the lower part the fibrous perichondrium is visible (HE×96)

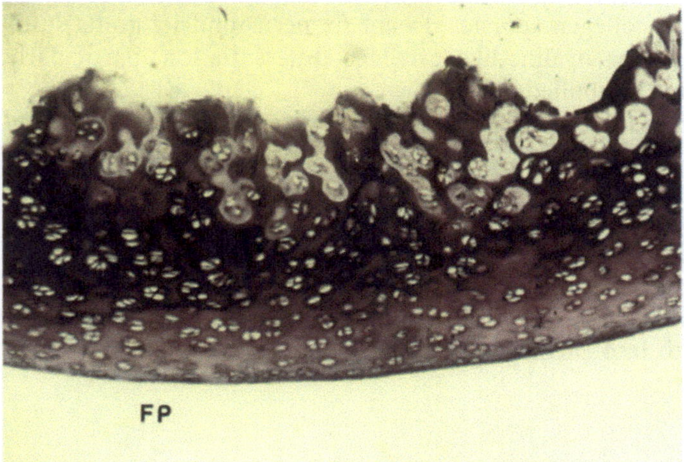

Fig. 5. Histochemical finding in perichondrial tissue after 14 days in culture [area between fibrous perichondrium (*FP*) and proliferation zone], The proliferation zone exhibits a strong staining of the hyalin ground substance, whereas the fibrous perichondrium does not show any staining (Toluidine Blue, pH 2.0, ×32)

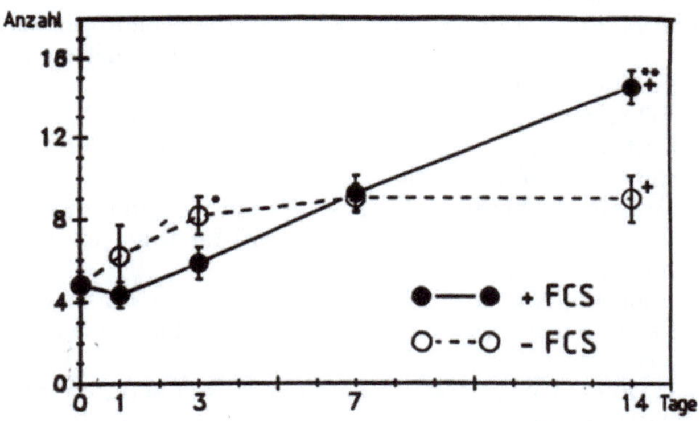

Fig. 6. Morphometric data of perichondrial culture (proliferation zone, number of isogenic groups). A distinct increase of the number of isogenic groups (chondrons) is detectable. (*FCS*, fetal calf serum; *single asterisk*, significant, or *double asterisks*, highly significant difference on the same day; *plus symbol*, significant difference in comparison to uncultured controls)

This means we observed no better cell differentiation, no improved fiber orientation of collagen fibers and no earlier production of ground substance. In comparison to fibrin glue fixation, the use of collagen sponges produced a detrimental effect. The quality of the junction between the graft, the subchondral bone and surrounding cartilage was poor. The gaps between graft and host were larger and did not show characteristics of enchondral ossification as seen in grafts with glue fixation. The explanation may be that collagen sponges do not fix perichondrial grafts sufficiently firmly to allow hyaline-like cartilage differentiation, particularly when active motion is applied.

Clinical investigations such as roentgenograms, magnetic resonance imaging or arthroscopy will have to demonstrate whether recommendations for postoperative conditions such as non-weight-bearing and CPM are transferable from experimental data into clinical practice. The advantages of perichondrial grafting for the repair of full thickness articular cartilage defects include the avoidance of immunological complications and the use of tissue that contains intrinsic proliferative potential to improve the ingrowth into cartilage defects.

References

Amiel D, Coutts RD, Abel M, Stewart W, Harwood F, Akeson WH (1985a) Rib perichondrial grafts for the repair of full-thickness articular-cartilage defects. J Bone Joint Surg 67A:911–920

Amiel D, Harwood FL, Abel MF, Akeson WH (1985b) Collagen types in neo-cartilage tissue resulting from rib perichondrial graft in an articular defect – a rapid semiquantitative methodology. Collagen Rel Res 5:337–347

Amiel D, Coutts RD, Harwood FL, Ishizue KK, Kleiner JB (1988) The chondrogenesis of rib perichondrial grafts for repair of full thickness articular cartilage defects in a rabbit model: a one year postoperative assessment. Conn Tissue Res 18:27–39

Bruns J, Kersten P, Lierse W, Silbermann M (1992) Autologous rib perichondrial grafts in experimentally induced osteochondral lesions in the sheep-knee joint: morphological results. Virchow Archiv A Pathol Anat 421:1–8

Bruns J, Kersten P, Lierse W, Weiss A, Silbermann M (1994) The in vitro influence of different culture conditions on the potential of sheep rib perichondrium to form hyaline-like cartilage. Virchow Archiv 424:169–175

Bulstra SK, Homminga GN, Buurman WA, Terwindt-Rouwenhorst E, van der Linden AJ (1990) The potential of adult human perichondrium to form hyalin cartilage in vitro. J Orthop Res 8:328–335

Coutts RD, Amiel D, Woo SL-Y, Akeson WH (1984) Technical aspects of perichondrial grafting in the rabbit. Eur Surg Res 16:322–328

Doerner (1798) De gravioribus quibusdam cartilaginum mutationibus. Tubingae. Cited by Mori M (1905) Studien über Knorpelregeneration. Dt Z Chir 76:220–234

Engkvist O, Ohlsen L (1979) Reconstruction of articular cartilage with free autologous perichondral grafts. Scand J Plast Reconstr Surg 13:269–274

Engkvist O, Skoog V, Pastacaldi P, Yormuk E, Juhlin R (1979) The cartilaginous potential of the perichondrium in rabbit ear and rib. Scand J Plast Reconstr Surg 13:275–280

Gaudernak T, Zifko B, Skorpik G (1986) Clinical experiences using fibrin sealant in the treatment of osteochondral fractures. In: Schlag G, Redl H (eds) Fibrin sealant in operative medicine, vol 7. Traumatology-Orthopedics. Springer, Berlin Heidelberg New York, pp 91–102

Homminga GN, van der Linden TJ, Terwindt-Rouwenhorst EAW (1989) Repair of articular defects by perichondrial grafts. Acta Orthop Scand 60:326–329

Homminga GN, Bulstra SK, Bouwmeester PM, van der Linden AJ (1990) Perichondrial grafting for cartilage lesions of the knee. J Bone Joint Surg 72B:1003–1007

Itay S, Abramovici A, Nevo Z (1987) The use of cultured embryonal chondrocytes as grafts for defects created in articular cartilage. Clin Orthop 220:270–279
Kaplonyi G, Zimmerman I, Frenyo AD, Farkas T, Emes G (1988) The use of fibrin adhesive in the repair of chondral and osteochondral injuries. Injury 19:267–272
Keller J, Andreassen TT, Joyce F, Knudsen VE, Jörgensen PH, Lucht U (1986) Biomechanical properties in osteochondral fractures fixed with fibrin sealant or kirschner wire. In: Schlag G, Redl H (eds) Fibrin sealant in operative medicine, vol 7. Traumatology-Orthopedics. Springer, Berlin Heidelberg New York, pp 86–90
Kimura T, Yasui N, Ohsawa S, Ono K (1984) Chondrocytes embedded in collagen gels maintain cartilage phenotype during long-term cultures. Clin Orthop 186:231–239
Kon M (1981) Cartilage formation from perichondrium in a weight-bearing joint. Eur Surg Res 13:387–396
Maor G, Mark K, Reddi H, Heinegard D, Franzen A, Silbermann M (1987) Acceleration of cartilage and bone formation on collagenous substrata. Collagen Rel Res 7:351–370
Ohlsen L, Widenfalk B (1983) The early development of articular cartilage after perichondrial grafting. Scand J Plast Reconstr Surg 17:163–177
Passl R, Plenk H, Sauer G, Spaengler HP, Radaszkiewicz T, Holle J (1976) Die reine homologe Gelenkknorpeltransplantation. Arch Orthop Unf-Chir 86:243–256
Pastacaldi P, Engkvist O (1979) Perichondrial wrist arthroplasty in rheumatoid patients. Hand 11:184–190
Salter RB, Simmonds DF, Malcolm BW, Rumble EJ, McMichael D (1975) The effects of continuous passive motion on the healing of articular cartilage defects. J Bone Joint Surg 57A:570–571
Salter RB, Simmonds DF, Malcolm BW, Rumble EJ, McMichael D, Clements ND (1980) The biological effect of continuous passive motion on the healing of full-thickness defects in articular cartilage. J Bone Joint Surg 62A:1232–1251
Schittek A, Demetriou AA, Seifter E, Stein JM, Levenson SM (1976) Microcrystalline collagen hemostat and wound healing. Ann Surg 184:697–704
Serradge H, Kutz JA, Kleinert HE, Lister GD, Wolff TW, Atasoy E (1984) Perichondrial resurfacing arthroplasty in the hand. J Hand Surg 9A:880–886
Skoog T, Ohlsen L, Sohn SA (1972) Perichondrial potential for cartilaginous regeneration. Scand J Plast Reconstr Surg 6:123–125
Skoog T, Ohlsen L, Sohn SA (1975) The chondrogenic potential of the perichondrium. Chir Plastica 3:91–103
Sully L, Jackson IT, Sommerland BC (1980) Perichondrial grafting in rheumatoid metacarpophalangeal joints. Hand 12:137–148
Tizzoni G (1878) Sulla istologia normale e patologica delle cartilagini ialine. Arch Sci Med 2:27–102
Upton J, Sohn SA, Glowacki J (1981) Neocartilage derived from transplanted perichondrium: what is it? Plast Reconstr Surg 68:166–172
Wakitani S, Kimura T, Hirooka A, Ochi T, Yoneda M, Yasui N, Owaki H, Ono K (1989) Repair of rabbit articular surfaces with allograft chondrocytes embedded in collagen gel. J Bone Joint Surg 71B:74–80
Woo SL-Y, Kwan M, Lee TQ, Field FP, Kleiner JB, Coutts RD (1987) Perichondrial autograft for the articular cartilage. Shear modulus of neocartilage studied in rabbits. Acta Orthop Scand 58:510–515
Yasui N, Osawa S, Ochi T, Nakashima H, Ono K (1982) Primary culture of chondrocytes embedded in collagen gels. Exp Cell Biol 50:92–100

Cartilage Destruction of the Knee Due to Partial Meniscal Resection

J. Grifka, T. Kalteis and W. Plitz

Introduction

Partial meniscal resection of the knee is the most frequent arthroscopic procedure. Statistical evaluations show that in more than 70% of the cases there is an isolated lesion of the posterior horn, due to trauma or degenerative changes. With sufficient arthroscopic skill, adequate equipment and appropriate instruments only the flap or damaged part is removed leaving a smooth and stable rest. We try to preserve as much meniscal tissue as possible and avoid damage to the cartilage of the femoral condyle or tibial plateau. Tears in the white/white or red/white area lacking healing potential, or painful degenerative tears are indications for resection. There is a biomechanical idea that mobile flaps or frayed edges may cause cartilage destruction due to interposition and shear motion. Reports about clinical outcome of the articular cartilage after meniscal resection are controversial.

Animal studies do not help because of different loading and moving situations in quadropedia. Therefore, we set up a standardized biomechanical test using fresh human cadaveric knee joints.

Experimental Set-Up

Different knee joint simulators have been developed for tribologic testing of knee endoprosthesis. We chose a testing machine that allows free motion in all six degrees of freedom and has no constraint, to enable us to create a gait-cycle with typical loading on the knee.

The knee joint simulator by Stallforth and Ungethüm (1977) fulfilled these requirements and could be adjusted to the cadaveric human knees with additional data accumulation like pressure measurements. To simulate a physiological loading, we programmed a gait-cycle according to Morrison (1968) and Seedhom and Hargreaves (1979). It had a double-step stress curve with a maximum load of 2000 N, considered to represent normal walking with highest pressure of the knee during heel-strike (calculated force as body weight multiple local velocity in axial loading of the bony structures).

Duration of the whole gait-cycle and bending of the specimens were standardized to match the physiologic situation. When reaching heel strike, the knee was slightly flexed at 20°. Within 190 ms full extension was achieved. Full ground contact of the foot stand phase lasted 300 ms, followed by toe-off, and then accelerated less loaded knee motion. The frequency was 0.85 Hz. This gait-cycle was continuously performed for 48 h.

We performed preliminary tests with 6 fresh knees before entering the definite study. This checked our correct testing conditions, including handling of the specimens, data registration and evaluation, and the cartilage condition during the trial.

We only accepted knees without any trauma or previous operation. The completely intact cartilage and meniscal condition was confirmed by arthroscopy (Fig. 1). The ligaments had to be completely intact. Radiological examination excluded bony changes. A knee was only accepted when the donor was within 20% range of the ideal Broca value of weight to body height. Our 24 specimens came from eight female and 16 male donors aged between 22 and 45 years (mean 31 years). They had died 36 to 48 h before testing.

The 18 knees for the definite trial were separated into three groups (I–III) consisting of six knees each. Series I formed the control group. After arthroscopic confirmation of completely intact cartilage surface and undisturbed meniscal status the knees were fixed in the testing device. They were covered by a transparent foil filled with Ringer's lactate solution and then immediately loaded under cyclic strain for 48 h (Figs. 2 and 3).

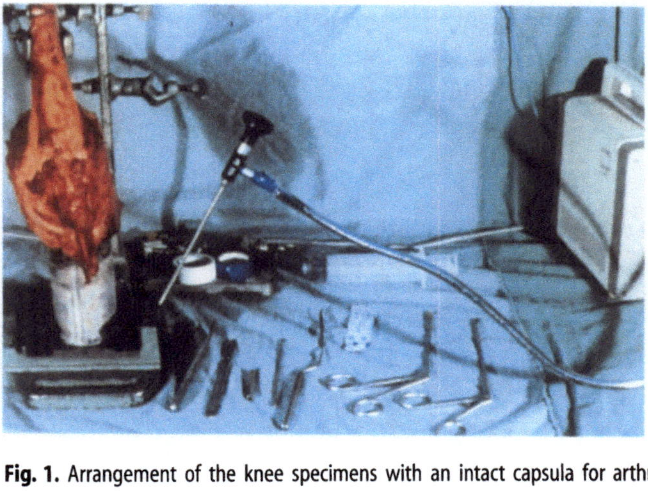

Fig. 1. Arrangement of the knee specimens with an intact capsula for arthroscopy

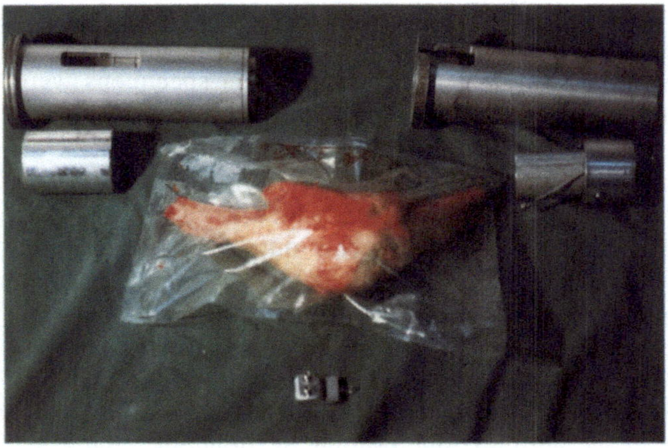

Fig. 2. Specimen covered with a foil (polyethylene) and surrounded by Purisole solution (sorbitol-mannitol). Tubes for femoral and tibial fixation in combination with pressure sonors

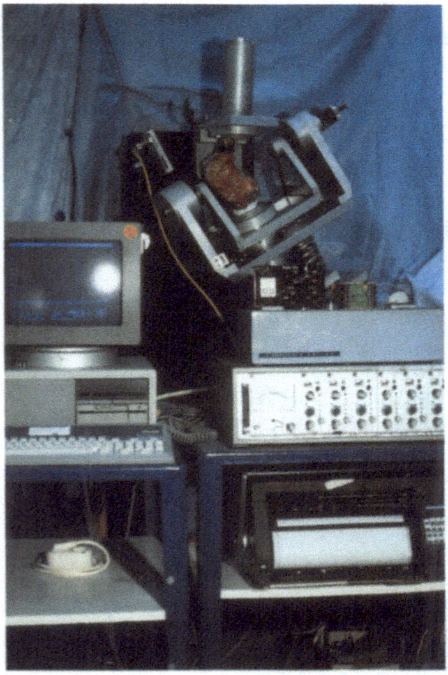

Fig. 3. Specimen fixed in the knee joint simulator by Stallforth and Ungethüm (1977) for gait-cycle movement and loading

In series II, the posterior horns of the medial and lateral menisci were incised arthroscopically, creating mobile flap lesions of about 2–2.5 cm length (Fig. 4). We checked that the flaps could interpose themselves into the knee joint line between femoral and tibial cartilage during flexion and extension.

For series III, arthroscopic partial resection of the posterior horns of the medial and lateral menisci was performed using a punch (Fig. 5). Attention was paid to establish a smooth, curved, stable rim.

After finishing the 48 h cyclic loading, ligaments and capsular structures were dissected and cartilage inspected. This included assessment and photodocumentation of the cartilage destruction according to Outerbridge (1961). Examination samples were preserved in 5% formalin solution for histology by light microscopy. Specimens were prepared for scanning electron microscope (SEM) analysis by soaking in 2.5% glutaraldehyde for at least 24 h and then in distilled water for another 24 h. Next, dehydration was performed using an increasing alcohol series. Then an increasing freon series was used before a final gold and coal application in vacuo.

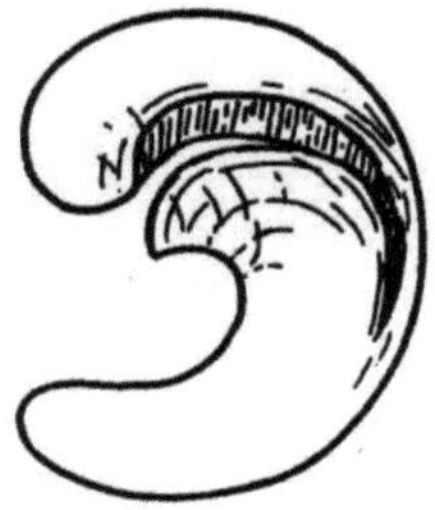

Fig. 4. Type of flap lesion at medial and lateral meniscus

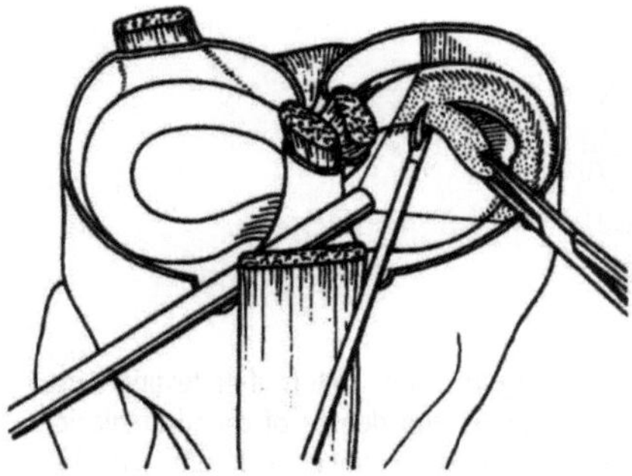

Fig. 5. Arthroscopic partial meniscal resection using three portals

Results

Immediately after testing gross differences could be seen macroscopically when dissecting the knees. The femoral condyles of the knees in series III showed severe destruction of at least Outerbridge grade III (Outerbridge 1961). In three knees grade IV changes were present, with bare bone lacking any cartilage coverage at certain spots. In contrast, in series I and II there was only mild cartilage alteration (Outerbridge Grade I, 1961). In one knee of series II, grade II was noticed. Overall there were no remarkable differences in the articular cartilage between the series with normal knee structures and those with mobile flap tears of the posterior meniscal horns after 48 h permanent cyclic moving and load bearing. In all six series III knees, we showed the presence of severe cartilage damage, mostly in the area that is in contact with the tibial plateau in about 40–60° flexion (Figs. 6–11).

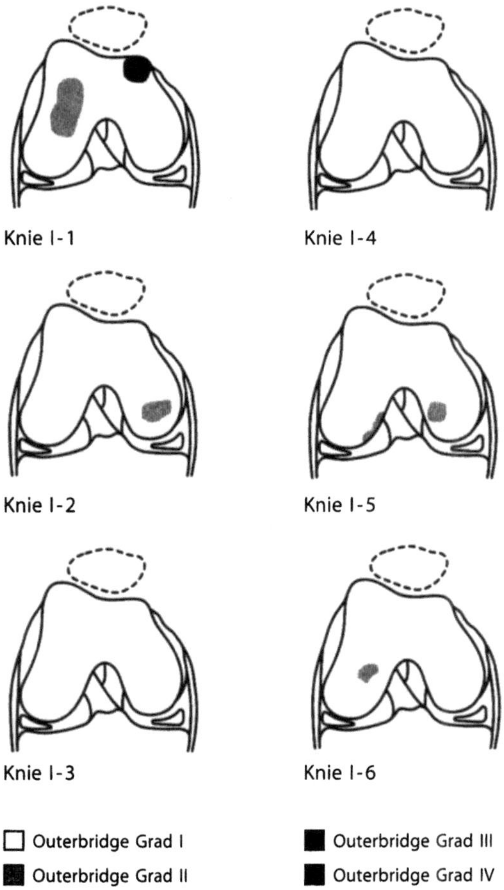

Fig. 6. Series I 48 h after testing. Localization and degree of chondromalacic changes according to Outerbridge (1961)

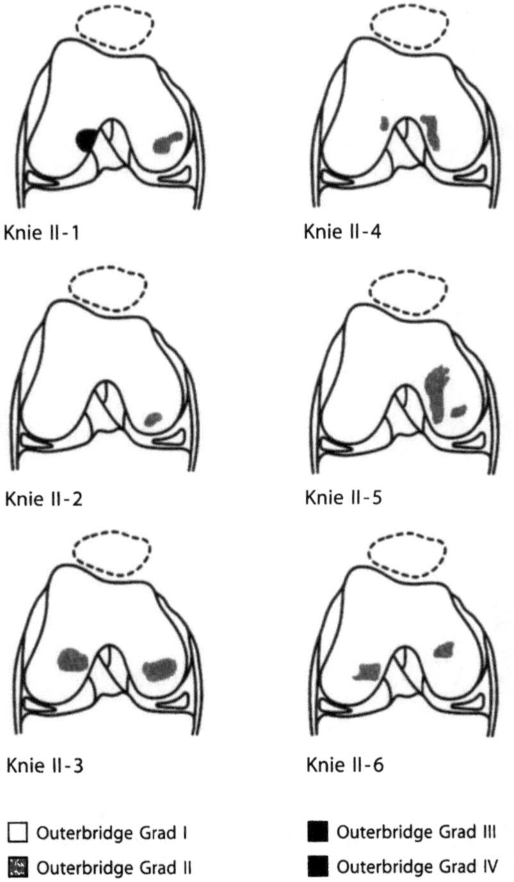

Fig. 7. Series II 48 h after testing. Localization and degree of chondromalacic changes according to Outerbridge (1961)

Histologic and SEM examination confirmed the macroscopic findings of severe damage in series III with the roughened joint surface. We saw bare cartilage fibers and the start of fibrillation at isolated spots in series II. In all knees the surrounding cartilage showed regular structure, chondrocyte distribution and nutritional supply.

During testing the roll-glide mechanism of group III changed. After about 12 h a remarkable translation motion between femur and tibia in those knees could be noticed, demonstrating instability. Correspondingly axial force transmission changed significantly compared to series I and II. After 24 h, the maximum force was diminished in series III, down to 46%. In series I and II the decrease was only 11% and 9%, respectively. A translational instability of these series was not detected.

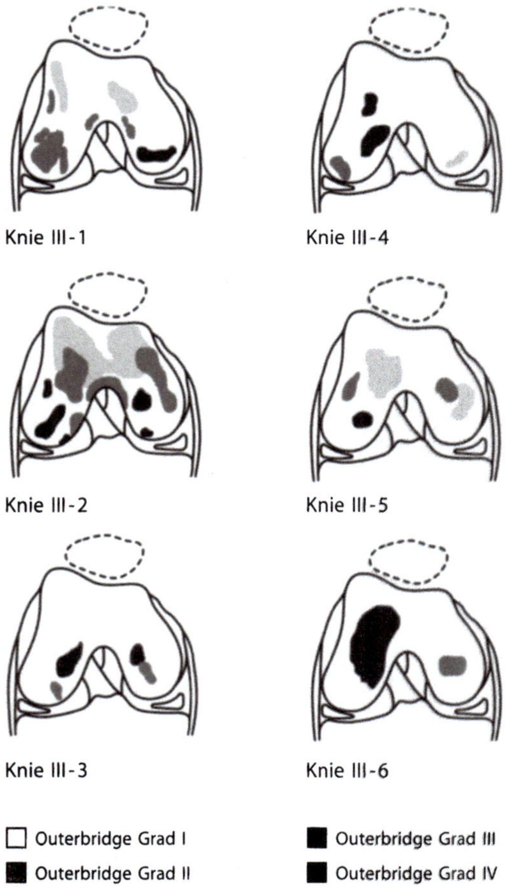

Fig. 8. Series III 48 h after testing. Localization and degree of chondromalacic changes according to Outerbridge (1961)

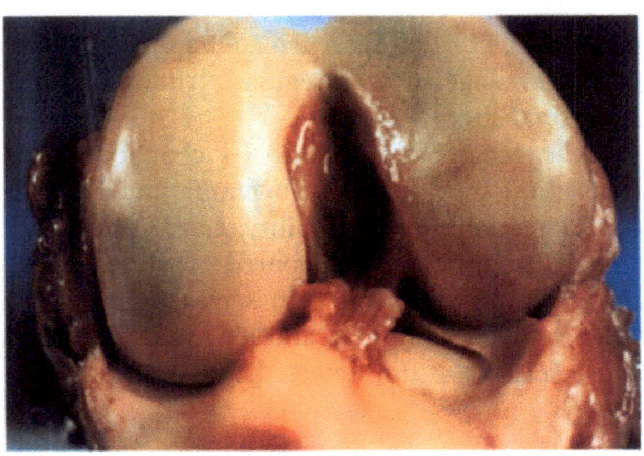

Fig. 9. Example of a specimen from series I (knee No. I-2) with original meniscal situation

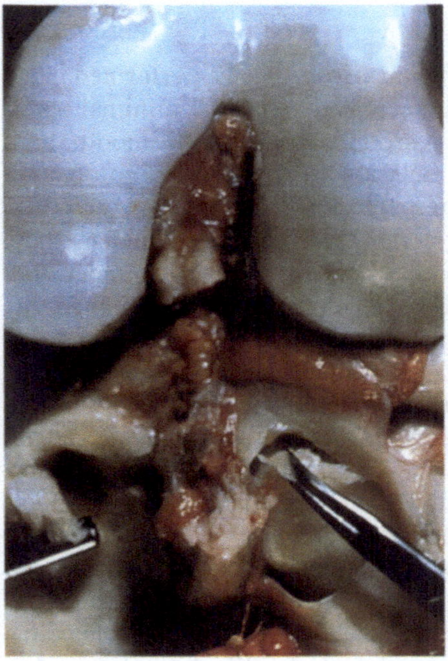

Fig. 10. Example of a specimen from series II (knee No. II-5) with mobile meniscal flap lesion medially and laterally

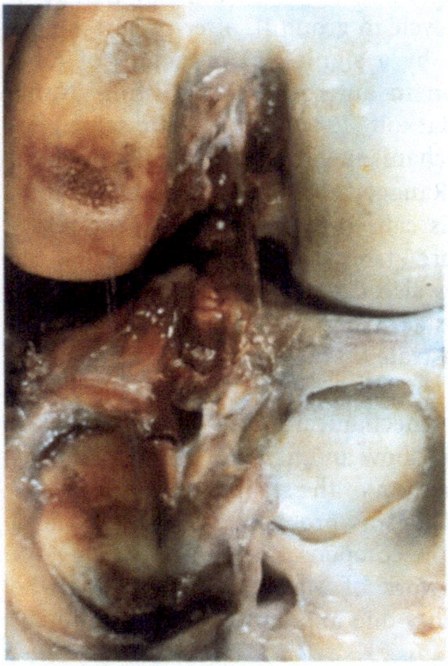

Fig. 11. Example of a specimen from series III (knee No. III-4) after partial meniscectomy of the posterior horns medially and laterally

Discussion

Induction of cartilage destruction after arthroscopically performed partial meniscus resection is not generally accepted. With the minimal invasive procedure and exact meniscal resection restoring a smooth and stable rim, we try to save meniscal function in stress distribution and knee motion. We evaluated the biomechanical risk of cartilage destruction following this intervention using a standardized test comparing partial resection and mobile flap tears with a control group with intact and regular cartilage. The biomechanical knee joint simulator designed by Stallforth and Ungethüm (1977) is a recognized tool for testing knee endoprostheses. Our special adjustments for human specimens include additional pressure registration at the bony shafts of the tibial and femoral fixation to calculate pressures in the knee and enables continuous control of forces while testing during 48 h. Strain causing unphysiologic stresses during flexion and extension was excluded due to the completely free motion of the knees in all six degrees of freedom. This allows motion pattern as determined by the bony contours and ligamentous structures.

To imitate a physiological bearing a gait-cycle with maximal compressive force of 2000 N was programmed. This load is above the forces calculated by Lindgren and Seireg (1989) using a computer model. We did not consider force moments of different muscles, but only the total amount of load directly on the knee joint. Excluding the complex mechanisms of physiological action between agonists and antagonists, we noted a major change of the role-glide mechanism during gait-cycle in group III after partial meniscus resection. This was accompanied by a significant reduction of force transmission and a visible translation in antero-postero shifting. Noble and Erat (1980) and Shoemaker and Markolf (1986) reported the same phenomenon of disturbed roll-gliding mechanism with abrupt displacement of the contact areas after meniscectomy. Rangger et al. (1994) assumed that an anterior and medial knee instability is caused by partial meniscus resection, although ligaments themselves are stable. Our study proves that the stabilizing function of the meniscus is also diminished in cases of partial meniscus resection in absence of the stabilizing muscle function.

Histologic and SEM analysis demonstrate that the local cartilage damage is not due to general changes such as softening or nutritional disturbance. This supports the hypothesis of pure mechanical abuse. Specimens with intact menisci or even mobile flap tears show an unchanged load transmission but a roll-gliding mechanism reduction of the stabilizing and load distributing function of the meniscus. This was probably due to the lack of additional active muscular stabilization compensating at least partly for the deficit. This corresponds to the work of Markolf et al. (1981) who found a ten times increased joint stability due to muscle contraction in ligamentous unstable knees.

Conclusion

The characteristic change of load distribution and disturbance of the roll-gliding mechanism even after partial meniscal resection in our biomechanical investigation demonstrates the importance of muscular stabilization in preventing or at least reducing cartilage destruction. This may also explain different outcomes after arthroscopic partial menisectomy in patients, depending on the amount of meniscus resected. Some of the poor results can be explained by inadequate muscular rehabilitation. The minor cartilage alterations in group II and the normal motion underlines the importance of the instability seen in group III. Of course, meniscus tears have to be resected due to pain and possible cartilage damage over a longer period of time.

References

Lindgren U, Seireg A (1989) The influence of the mediolateral deformity, tibial torsion and foot position on femortibial load. Arch Orthop Trauma Surg 108:22–26

Markolf KL, Bargar WL, Shoemaker SC, Amstutz HC (1981) The role of joint load in knee stability. J Bone Surg 63A:570–585

Morrison JB (1968) Bioengineering analysis of force actions transmitted by the knee joint. Bio Med Eng 3:164–170

Noble J, Erat K (1980) In defense of the meniscus. A prospective study of 200 meniscectomy patients. J Bone Joint Surg 62B:7–11

Outerbridge RE (1961) The etiology of chondromalacia patellae. J Bone Joint Surg 43B:752-757

Rangger C, Glotzer W, Benedetto KP (1994) Ligament instability after arthroscopic partial medial meniscus resection. Unfallchirurg 97:435–437

Shoemaker, Markolf KL (1986) The role of the menisci in the anterior-posterior stability of the loaded anterior cruciate-deficient knee. J Bone Joint Surg 68:71–79

Seedhom BB, Hargreaves DJ (1979) Transmission of the load in the knee joint with special reference to the role of the menisci. Part II: Experimental results, discussion and conclusion. Eng Med 8:220–228

Stallforth H, Ungethüm M (1977) Entwicklung eines Kniegelenksimulators. Arch Orthop Unfall-Chir 90:343–353

Meniscus Replacement and Osteoarthrosis

D. Lazovic

Introduction

After Broadhurst first described the meniscectomy in 1866, total resection of the meniscus was used for all meniscal lesions (Wirth et al. 1988). Even in 1978 Smilie proposed this as the therapy of choice, although more understanding of meniscal functions followed (Smilie 1978). McGinty demonstrated the advantages of a partial resection in a large study in 1977 (McGinty et al. 1977). Trying to preserve as much meniscus tissue as possible logically led to the concept of meniscal repair (Wirth 1981). This is now the current thinking.

Understanding the multiple functions of the meniscus and the necessity for preservation, another possible avenue of exploration was to replace the meniscus after its total loss by injury or previous operation. Homologous transplants, prostheses or tendinous substitutes have been tried (Milachowski et al. 1987; Toyonaga et al. 1983; Kohn 1989).

Functions of the Meniscus

The main function of the meniscus seems to be load transmission (Fairbank 1948; Seedhom and Hargreaves 1979) and, associated with this, shock absorption (Voloshin and Wosk 1983). The meniscus plays an important role in knee joint stabilization especially with loss of the anterior cruciate ligament (Hsieh and Walker 1976). Other functions are lubrication of the joint and nutrition of the cartilage (McConaill 1932; Webber et al. 1986). All this results in the meniscus playing a major role in the prevention of knee joint osteoarthritis (Fairbank 1948).

The meniscus distributes load to a larger area. Load transmission mainly takes place in the medial and dorsal meniscus-covered area and moves further back with knee flexion (Fukabayshi and Kurosawa 1980; Kettelkamp and Jacobs 1972; Krause et al. 1976; Kurosawa et al. 1980; Shrive et al. 1978; Walker and Erkmann 1975). The axial load is transformed to circular hoop stress in order to relieve the strain on the tibial surface (Kummer 1994; Shrive et al. 1978) (Fig. 1a).

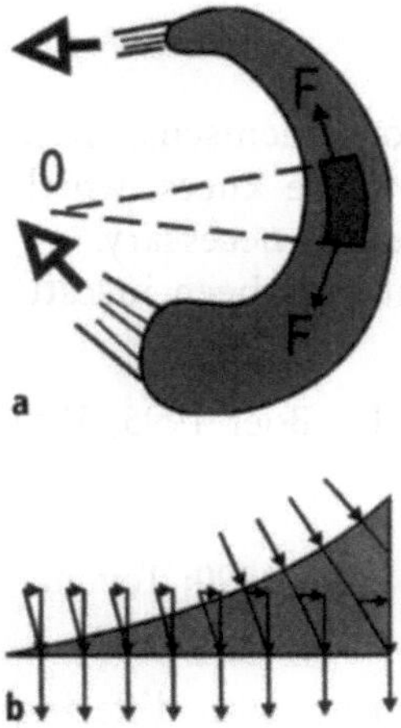

Fig. 1. a The meniscus transforms the load to circumferential forces (*F*), which are transmitted to the anterior and posterior attachments (*arrows*). The direction of forces is approximately perpendicular to the radius of a virtual center of the knee (*O*). **b** The meniscus takes up forces perpendicular to its surface and distributes them to axial forces on the tibial plateau and centrifugal forces, that push the meniscus peripherally

The resulting forces of the femoral condyle are inclined to the tibia but perpendicular to the meniscal surface. These forces can be divided into vectors vertical and parallel to the tibia, the latter pushing the meniscus peripherally out of the joint (Fig. 1b). This is counteracted by the circular located fibrous structures and the ligamentous insertions of the meniscus (Shrive et al. 1978). An intact circular structure therefore seems to be the condition for perfect function of the meniscus as a load transmitter (Kohn 1989; Kummer 1994; Mow et al. 1992; Shrive et al. 1978). Partial or total meniscectomy allows up to threefold an increase in peak stresses (Krause et al. 1976; Kurosawa et al. 1980; Shrive et al. 1978).

Shock-absorption is supported by the biphasic properties of the meniscus, taking in water unloaded and relieving it under load (Zhu et al. 1994). Shock-absorption is 20% greater with an intact meniscus than in knees without (Hoshino and Wallace 1989; Voloshin and Wosk 1983).

Stabilization of the knee joint is primarily provided by the ligaments, but the meniscus acts as a secondary stabilizer. Loss of the medial meniscus does not increase antero-posterior motion, but will still lead to an anterior and medial instability with time (Rangger et al. 1994; Sonne-Holm et al. 1981). In knees deficient in the anterior cruciate ligament, the amount of instability will be one third higher with medial meniscectomy (Hsieh and Walker 1976; Levy et al. 1982). Instability could also be due to a vacuum effect because the thin fluid film between the meniscus and the joint surface causes adhesion forces that are reduced even with slight incongruency. Meniscectomy has been shown to disturb proprioception (Müller 1994).

Osteoarthrosis is the main consequence of loss of the meniscal functions and is directly related to the amount of meniscal tissue removed (Cox et al. 1975; Fairbank 1948).

Meniscus Replacement

In spite of attempts to preserve or reconstruct the torn meniscus, there are still some indications for total meniscectomy. In these knees, which usually have multiple pathology, a meniscus replacement is necessary.

Three different techniques for meniscal replacement have been investigated:

1. Allografts (Milachowski et al. 1987; Van Arkel and De Boer 1995; Verdonk et al. 1994)
2. Autografts (Kohn 1989)
3. Prosthesis (Kenny et al. 1983; Messner 1994; Stone et al. 1990; Toyonaga et al. 1983).

Allografts and autografts have been used in clinical trials with differing results (Milachowski et al.; Van Arkel and De Boer 1995; Verdonk et al. 1994). Prostheses are mainly used in animal experiments, but the first series with a collagen scaffold is now under investigation (Messner 1994; Sommerlath and Gillquist 1992; Stone et al. 1992; Toyonaka et al. 1983). The mechanical properties of the graft have the best results in allogenic transplants (Sommerlath and Gillquist 1992). But in all meniscus replacements there are still some disadvantages: the allogenic transplant has to be sterilised to avoid viral transmission (especially HIV), and autologous tissue lacks mechanical properties as do prostheses (Kohn 1989; Sommerlath and Gillquist 1992).

For all replacements the effect of incongruity or an isometric placement on the cartilage is unknown. The following questions need to be answered:

1. What happens if the load transmission is altered by the incongruous surfaces of meniscal grafts?
2. Does it disturb the transmission of axial load to centrifugal forces (Fig. 2a)?
3. Does the malpositioning of the ligamentous insertions disturb the transformation of load into hoop stresses (Fig. 2b)?

Methods

We used an experimental animal study to investigate the effects of incongruency or anisometricity of meniscal grafts on the knee joint cartilage. Operations were performed on 30 knees of fully grown Black-Head sheep. They were randomly divided into five groups (Table 1).

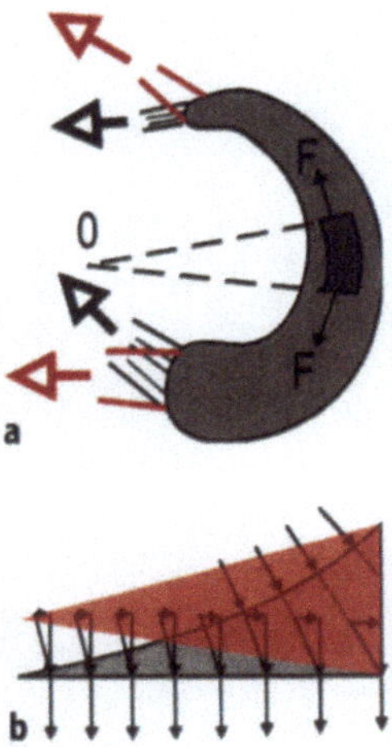

Fig. 2. a A displacement of the tibial attachments of the meniscus can lead to an altered load transmission despite an anatomical correct position of the meniscal body itself. **b** An incongruity of the meniscal surfaces can lead to altered force (*F*) distribution in the meniscus and therefore change the load transmission. *O*, virtual center of the knee

Table 1. Study groups

Group	Surgical Technique	Number of knees
1	Non-operated	5
2	Sham-operation	5
3	Total medial meniscectomy	10
4	Incongruous graft	5
5	Anisometric graft	5

Study Groups

The study groups consisted of three control and two test groups. For control we used the following:

1. five non-operated knees;
2. five sham-operated knees. In this group a standardized medial approach was used. The joint was opened medially with detachment of the medial collateral ligament, which was refixed after the intraarticular procedure by a cancellous screw. In this group the medial meniscus was totally dissected from the capsule and refixed in place. This provided us with data on the effect of the operative approach, which could itself lead to cartilage alterations caused by instability due to the detachment of the medial collateral ligament or by meniscal changes due to disturbed blood supply (Jackson et al. 1992) (Fig. 3a).
3. Ten meniscectomised knees. This provided data on osteoarthritis induced by total medial meniscectomy that had to be improved by meniscus grafts in the other groups.

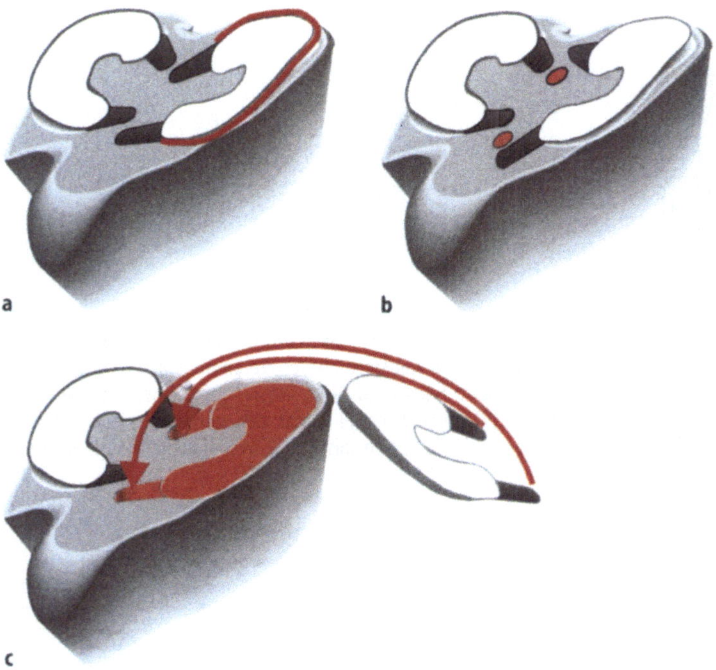

a b c

Fig. 3. **a** The sham-operation. The meniscus was totally dissected from the capsule and then refixed in place with four absorbable sutures. The mechanical functions of the attachments remained unchanged (*red line*, line of dissection). **b** The incongruity operation. After a total meniscectomy the meniscus of the contralateral knee was implanted with regard to the correct anatomical insertions. The meniscal ligaments were reattached through tibial bone tunnels. This resulted in unchanged shape and position of the meniscus, just creating an incongruity of the surfaces. **c** The anisometric operation. After total meniscectomy the meniscus was replaced anatomically with displaced drill holes for the anterior and posterior attachments. This created anisometric conditions (*red*, anatomic position of anterior and posterior ligamentous insertion)

The operative technique of the test groups should lead to an incongruous or to an anisometric meniscus replacement.

4. Five knees with an incongruous meniscus. With the standardized medial approach the medial meniscus was totally dissected. The medial meniscus of the contra-lateral side was implanted using the original insertion points without displacement and refixed to the capsule with four absorbable sutures. The ligamentous attachments of the anterior and posterior horn were refixed by transosseous anchoring sutures through drill holes, placed with an aiming device. Using this technique with the contra-lateral meniscus, we had a graft with the symmetric proportions of the original meniscus, not changing the circumferential tension. Length, curvature and thickness were the same. Only the surfaces were exchanged from the femoral condyle to the tibial plateau; thus creating an incongruency (Fig. 3b).

5. Five knees with anisometric placement of the anterior and posterior meniscal insertions. Again using the standardized medial approach the medial meniscus was totally dissected. Afterwards it was refixed with the meniscus body remaining in place but the anterior and posterior ligaments were refixed through anchoring drill holes displaced anteriorly or posteriorly to the original insertions. This was feasible as the anterior and posterior attachment ligaments of the meniscus were 4–6 mm, which allowed transposition of the attachments without movement of the body. The meniscus body itself was refixed with four absorbable sutures. This led to a congruous meniscus, unchanged in position, but with a diversion of the hoop stresses and diminished circular tension (Fig. 3 c).

Evaluation

After 24 weeks the knee joint was retrieved and cartilage alterations were evaluated by microscopic and macroscopic criteria. For evaluation, all knees were photographed with a scale after retrieval. The surface size and insertion places were measured by digital analysis software (Optimas 5.0). Gross examination of the meniscus and the underlying cartilage was graded as described by Jackson et al. (1992) (Table 2). For histological evaluation of the cartilage, biopsy samples (3 mm×15 mm) were taken at standard locations corresponding to the anterior, midle and posterior parts of the meniscus. They were fixed, decalcified and stained with Safranin-O fast green iron (SOFG), which is an acknowledged standardized technique for evaluation of osteoarthritis (Mankin 1971). It assesses the cartilage degeneration by changes in the cartilage structure, cell changes, reaction to SOFG staining and integrity of the tidemark (Table 3). The data were analysed with the non-parametric Mann and Whitney U-test.

Table 2. Criteria for morphologic assessment of cartilage changes according to Jackson et al. (1992)

Grade	Morphologic appearance
1	Intact surface, color changes or loss of cartilage, no bone exposition
2	Surface fibrillation or loss of cartilage, no bone exposition
3	Less than 10% of bone exposition in given region
4	More than 10% of bone exposition, fragmentation of cartilage around the lesion

Table 3. Criteria for histologic assessment of cartilage changes according to Mankin et al. (1971)

1.	**Structure**	**Grade**
a	Normal	0
b	Surface irregularities	1
c	Pannus and surface irregularities	2
d	Clefts to transitional zone	3
e	Clefts to radial zone	4
f	Clefts to calcified zone	5
g	Complete disorganization	6
2.	**Cells**	**Grade**
a	Normal	1
b	Diffuse hypercellularity	2
c	Cloning	3
d	Hypocellularity	4
3.	**Safranin-O staining**	**Grade**
a	Normal	0
b	Slight reduction	1
c	Moderate reduction	2
d	Severe reduction	3
e	No dye noted	4
4.	**Tidemark integrity**	**Grade**
a	Intact	0
b	Crossed by blood vessels	1

Results

Meniscus Morphology

No changes were seen in the untreated group 1. On average the medial meniscus covered an area of 3.97 cm^2, that is 53% of the medial tibial plateau.

In the sham-operated group 2 all menisci healed to the capsule. Only one meniscus showed slight irregularities in the mid portion. All the others were unchanged. The average area covered was 4.07 cm^2 (55%).

In group 3, the medial meniscectomy group, three meniscus-like regenerative structures were seen, one of them reaching an area of 3.33 cm^2, but mainly much smaller or without rebuild tissue. The mean coverage was 22% of the medial tibial plateau.

In group 4, where the menisci were incongruous, changes were obvious. The menisci had superficial irregularities and revealed changes in color. But no ruptures or dislocations occurred. The shape adapted to the femoral and tibial surfaces, so that it was flat to the tibial plateau and concave to the femoral condyle. The mean covered area of 4.70 cm^2 (51%) resembled that of an intact meniscus.

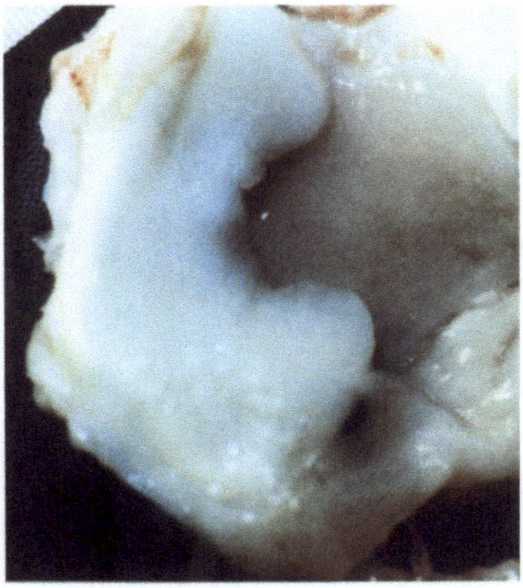

Fig. 4. Example of a meniscus of the anisometric group. Most menisci suffered substantial loss, but none was displaced or disrupted

In group 5 with an anisometric attachment of the menisci, the worst changes were seen. The menisci showed substantial loss, covering on average an area of only 40% (3.34 cm^2), but no disruption or dislocation of the attachments was seen (Fig. 4).

Tibial Morphology

In group 1, as expected no changes were seen. All cartilage surfaces seemed smooth and undamaged so they were graded as 0 according to Jackson.

In group 2, the sham operation showed only a color change of the cartilage, but no fibrillation and was graded with a mean of 0.5.

In group 3, the meniscectomy led to intense damage with fibrillation and even cartilage loss to the bone. Osteophytes were formed. The degree of degeneration was 1.7.

Color changes and fibrillation, but no cartilage loss were seen in group 4, with incongruous meniscal transplants. The average grade of changes was 1.3 (Fig. 5).

Severe damage to the cartilage was seen in group 5. The menisci with displaced attachments had caused fibrillation and major cartilage loss, graded 2.6 (Fig. 6).

No differences were seen in the non-operated and the sham-operated knees. The results of the morphologic assessment of all other groups were significantly different from these two. The meniscectomy group was slightly inferior compared to the incongruous meniscus group but better than the group with displaced attachments. However, these differences were not statistically significant (Fig. 7, Table 4).

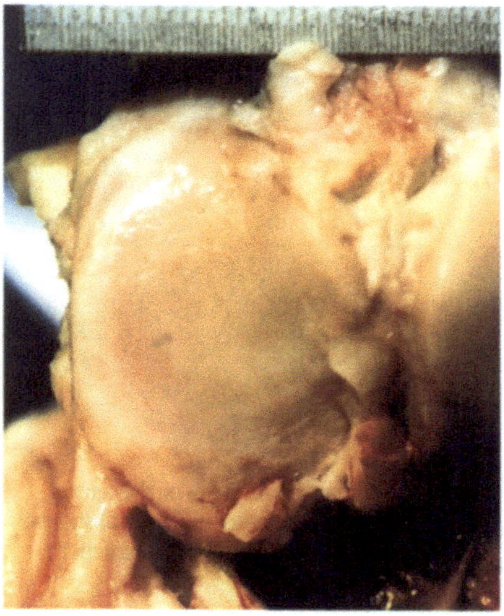

Fig. 5. Example of tibial plateau changes after incongruous meniscus replacement

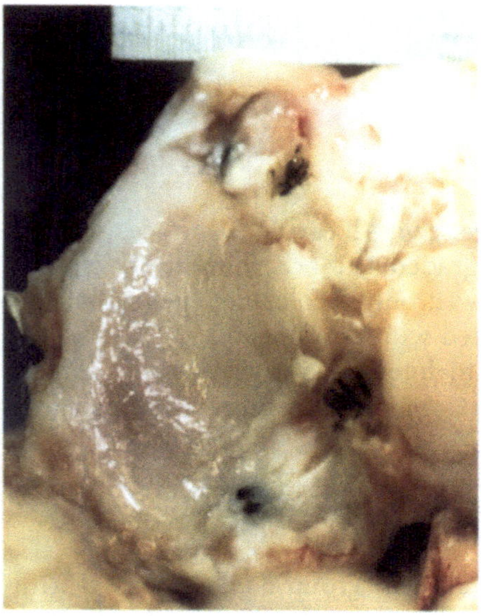

Fig. 6. Example of tibial plateau changes after anisometric meniscus replacement

Using the digital analysis program we were able to measure the coverage of the tibial plateau by the meniscus and the exact amount of displacement of the anterior and posterior insertion points of the menisci (Table 5). With a very low standard deviation the anterior insertion was displaced by 8.6 mm and the posterior insertion by 11.2 mm (Table 5).

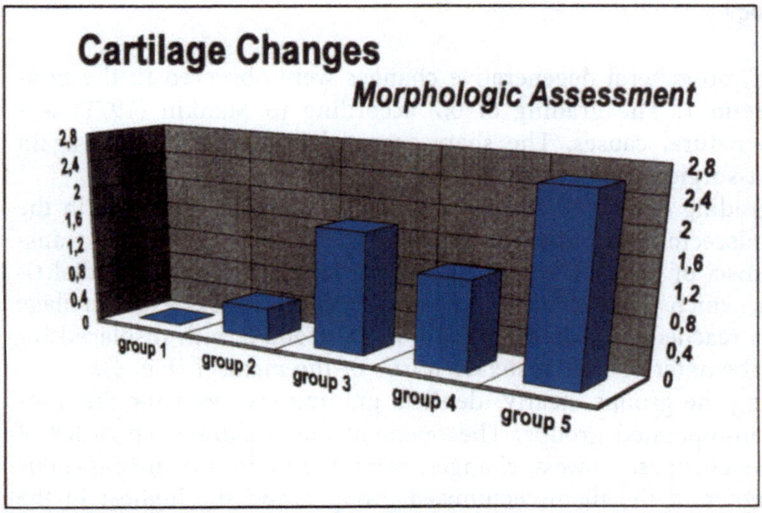

Fig. 7. Data of the morphologic assessment. *group 1*, Non-operated knees; *group 2*, sham-operated knees; *group 3*, meniscectomised knees; *group 4*, knees with an incongruous meniscal graft; *group 5*, knees with an anisometric meniscal graft. Grading according to Jackson et al. (1992)

Table 4. Overall results for morphologic and histologic assessment of tibial cartilage changes

Group	Treatment	Morphologic grading	Histologic grading
1	Non-operated	0	0.7
2	Sham-operated	0.46	0.6
3	Meniscectomy	2.2	6.0
4	Incongruous meniscus	2.0	4.1
5	Anisometric meniscus	2.6	8.0

Table 5. Data from the digital image analysis for the coverage of the tibial plateau by the meniscus

Group	Tibial plateau (cm^2)	Meniscus (cm^2)	Coverage (%)
1	7.48	3.97	53%
2	7.35	4.04	55%
3	8.91	1.95	22%
4	8.99	4.60	51%
5	8.40	3.34	40%

Tibial Histology

As expected, no general degenerative changes were observed in the non-operated group 1. The grading of 0.7 according to Mankin (1971) was ascribed to natural causes. The sham-operated knees of group 2 again showed post-surgical changes graded 0.6.

A high grading of 6 for the medial tibial compartment was seen in the medial meniscectomised knees of group 3. The incongruously transplanted menisci of group 4 led to cartilage degeneration of the medial tibial plateau, which was graded 4.1. Again, the highest degree of cartilage damage was reached with an average of 8.0 in group 5 with displaced insertions of the anterior and posterior horns of the menisci (Fig. 8).

Comparing the groups, nearly identical grading was seen for the non- and the sham-operated groups. The operated knees showed an order of degenerative changes. Lowest changes were found in the incongruous group 4, higher in the meniscectomised group 3 and the highest in the group 5 with displaced attachments of the meniscus (Fig. 9). These differences were statistically significant.

The operative approach seemed to have little influence on cartilage damage and the meniscus did not seem to suffer from capsular dissection and refixation. The use of an incongruous meniscus as a transplant

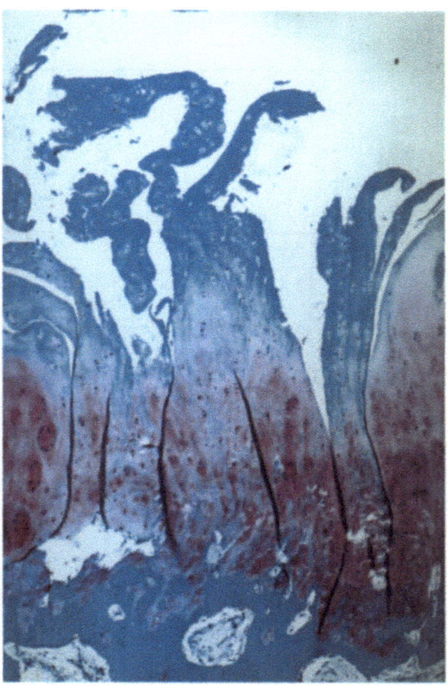

Fig. 8. Example of histological changes of the tibial cartilage after anisometric meniscus replacement

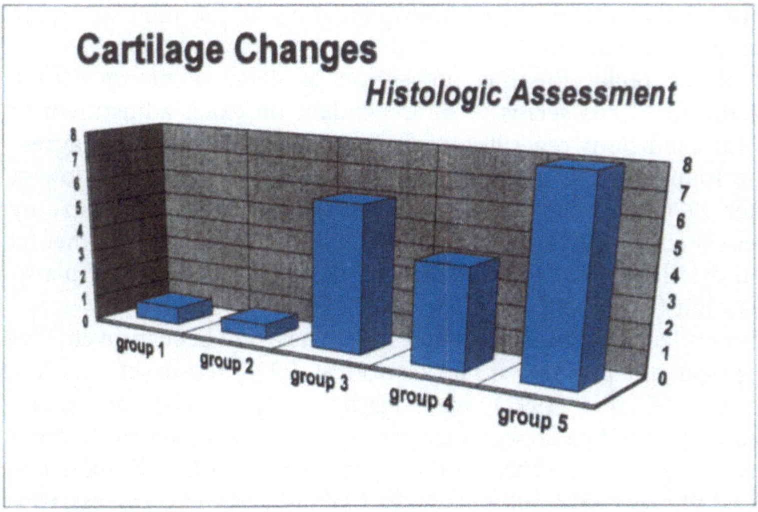

Fig. 9. Histologic assessment. *group 1,* Non-operated knees; *group 2,* sham-operated knees; *group 3,* meniscectomised knees; *group 4,* knees with an incongruous meniscal graft; *group 5,* knees with an anisometric meniscal graft. Grading according to Mankin et al. (1971)

led to osteoarthritic changes but had still some chondroprotective effect compared to meniscectomy. The use of a meniscus suitable in size and shape but not attached to the isometric insertion points will lead to an even worse osteoarthritis than a total meniscectomy.

Discussion

Meniscus replacement can be done with autogenous tissue, allogenic transplants and alloplastic prostheses. Although all have been used clinically, indications and operative techniques vary for these materials (Arnoczky and Milachowski 1990; Jackson et al. 1992; Kohn 1989; Milachowski et al. 1988; Milachowski et al. 1989; Sommerlath and Gillquist 1992). The suggested indications are: total loss of meniscus in the younger patient, destroyed medial meniscus with loss of the anterior cruciate ligament, varus gonarthritis grade I and marked varus gonarthritis of older patients (Arnoczky and Milachowski 1990; Milachowski et al. 1988; Stone et al. 1990; Van Arkel and De Boer 1995; Verdonk et al. 1994; Wirth et al. 1988; Zukor et al. 1990). Various operative techniques have been used: replacement only of the meniscal body with suture fixation at the capsule, suture fixation at still available anterior and posterior insertion ligaments, fixation of the anterior and posterior ligament with bone blocks of different kinds, and even transplantation of the meniscus with the underlying tibial plateau.

The aim of the replacement is prevention or delay of osteoarthritis. Function of the meniscus seems to be dependent on exact adjustment to the anatomical conditions regarding material, size and fixation. No agreement can be found on the material with the best properties and lowest risk (Messner 1994). Selection of a transplant by determining the size by magnetic resonance imaging seems meaningful but is still experimental (Arnoczky and Milachowski 1990). Not much is known about ideal placement and fixation (Kohn and Moreno 1994).

Meniscectomy leads to osteoarthritis, but it has not been proven that meniscus replacement prevents it (Jackson et al. 1992; Moon, et al. 1988; Sommerlath and Gillquist 1992). Investigations rely on clinical experience. Experimental studies concentrate more on the effect on the meniscus itself (Arnoczky et al. 1990; Canham and Stanish 1986; Kohn 1989; Milachowski et al. 1987; Milachowski et al. 1989; Shelton and Dukes 1994; Sommerlath and Gillquist 1992; Van Arkel and De Boer 1995; Verdonk et al. 1994; Wirth et al. 1988).

Thus, in our study we concentrated on the effects of incongruency and displaced insertion in the tibial cartilage. Our control groups gave us the basic data for comparison with the test groups. The operative approach did not affect the tibial cartilage insignificantly. The medial meniscus healed to the capsule in all cases and showed no degenerative changes. No dislocation occurred in spite of the minimal refixation to the capsule with only four absorbable sutures. The attachment to the anterior and posterior insertion was probably more important than the capsular attachment. It seemed that the operative approach did influence the cartilage but did not damage it. As the approach was standardized for all other procedures, we were able to compare their data with our control group 2.

The medial meniscectomy was the model that had to be improved by meniscus replacement. As expected it showed a high amount of osteoarthritis in macroscopic and microscopic assessment. Although regenerative tissue formed, which could gain size and some macroscopic aspects of an intact meniscus, it could not prevent osteoarthritic changes. This substitute could not restore meniscal function. The grade of osteoarthritis was independent of its size.

In our test group 4, with incongruous meniscus transplants, significant osteoarthritis occurred, but it was still less than in the meniscectomised group. To transform axial load into circumferential stresses, the femoral condyle and tibial plateau has to have contact with the meniscus to transmit pressure (Fairbank 1948; Kohn 1989). We investigated whether incongruency of the meniscus has an influence on the cartilage. The operative technique provided anatomical positioning of the anterior and posterior insertions. The hoop stresses should remain unchanged. Still osteoarthritis occurred. Explanations could be that the incongruency had a negative effect on lubrication and nutrition. Also, it is known that the mechanical properties of the meniscus vary within itself (Zhu et al. 1994). Probably the load transmission could not work to the necessary degree of sophistication. Other authors have reported on lengthening of the ligamentous insertions, which could affect the isotonic conditions of load transmission (Gao and Messner 1996). Still the influence of incongruency is low. Taking size, volume and anatomical isotonic positioning of the insertions into account, it can obviously meet the requirements of load transmission and transformation. Compared with total medial meniscectomy, it prevented osteoarthritis.

In meniscus transplantation the correct placement for anterior and posterior insertions has to be selected. As little is known about the ideal localization of the insertions, it seems likely that isotonic conditions are not reproducible. We investigated this in group 5 by choosing non-anatomical insertions. This led to the worst osteoarthritic changes in our study. The meniscus seems to get mechanically destroyed; thus, creating more forces on the tibial plateau rather than protecting it. The results suggest that displacement of the anterior and posterior attachments decreases the ability of the meniscus to transform axial load to circumferential hoop stress. The mere volume of the meniscus body interposing between femoral condyle and tibial plateau has no preventing effect on osteoarthritis. This could be expected as Seedhom and Hargreaves had already stated in 1979 that a stable and elastic attachment is necessary to transform vertical forces into circular tension and an elongation will lead to a dysfunction of the meniscus (Seedhom and Hargreaves 1979). The importance of the insertion placement for meniscus replacement of all kinds was pointed out by Kohn (1989). Our study shows that a meniscus transplant whose insertions are displaced will lead to even more cartilage destruction than total meniscectomy despite being of ideal size and shape.

Conclusions

Meniscal replacement could prevent or delay osteoarthritis in a meniscus deficient knee. Of critical importance for achieving this aim is the reconstruction of the meniscal functions. The main requirement is the ability to transform the axial load to circumferential stress. Our study suggests that isometric positioning of the meniscal attachments is as important for the meniscal function as it is for the anterior cruciate in ligament reconstruction. Neglecting this, a meniscus replacement will lead to more osteoarthritis than a total meniscectomy. Incongruency of the replacement seems of less importance as long as the insertions are chosen correctly.

1. Meniscus replacements can re-establish load distribution (Paletta et al. 1997).
2. The insertions are essential for load distribution (Seedhom and Hargreaves 1979).
3. Non-anatomic insertions induce osteoarthritis.
4. Congruity is less important than insertion position.
5. An isometric and congruous meniscal graft will prevent or delay osteoarthritis.

References

Arnoczky SP, Milachowski KA (1990) Meniscal allografts: where do we stand? In: Ewing JW (ed) Articular cartilage and knee joint function: basic science and arthroscopy. Raven Press, New York, pp 129–136

Arnoczky SP, Warren RF, McDevitt CA (1990) Meniscal replacement using a cryopreserved allograft. Clin Orthop 252:121–128

Canham W, Stanish W (1986) A study of the biological behavior of the meniscus as a transplant in the medial compartment of a dog's knee. Am J Sports Med 14:376–379

Cox JS, Nye CE, Schaefer WW, Woodstein IJ (1975) The degenerative effects of partial and total resection of the medial meniscus in dogs' knees. Clin Orthop 109:178–183

Fairbank TJ (1948) Knee joint changes after meniscectomy. J Bone Joint Surg 30B:664–670

Fukubayashi T, Kurosawa H (1980) The contact area and pressure distribution pattern of the knee. Acta Orthop Scand 51:871–879

Gao J, Messner K (1996) Natural healing of anterior and posterior attachments of the rabbit meniscus. Clin Orthop 328:276–284

Hoshino A, Wallace HA (1989) Impact absorbing properties of the human knee joint. J Jpn Orthop Ass 63:67–74

Hsieh H, Walker PS (1976) Stabilizing mechanisms of the loaded and unloaded knee joint. J Bone Joint Surg 58A:87–93

Jackson DW, McDevitt CA, Simon TM, Arnoczky SP, Atwell EA, Silvino NJ (1992) Meniscal transplantation using fresh and cryopreserved allografts. An experimental study in goats. Am J Sports Med 20:644–656

Kenny C, Krackow KA, McCarthy EF (1983) An evaluation of the effects of a silastic meniscus prosthesis in postmeniscectomy osteoarthritis. Trans 29th Annual ORS Meeting 8:335

Kettelkamp DB, Jacobs AW (1972) Tibiofemoral contact area, determination and implications. J Bone Joint Surg 54A:349–356

Kohn D (1989) Der plastische Ersatz des Innenmeniskus mit körpereigenem Gewebe, eine experimentelle Untersuchung. Hannover, Med. Hochsch, Habil.-Schr

Kohn D, Moreno B (1994) Meniskusinsertion. Orthopäde 23:98–101

Krause WR, Pope MH, Johnson RJ, Wilder DG (1976) Mechanical changes in the knee after meniscectomy. J Bone Joint Surg 58A:599–607

Kummer B (1994) Biomechanik des Meniskus. Orthopäde 23:90–92

Kurosawa H, Fukubayashi T, Nakajima H (1980) Load-bearing mode of the knee joint: physical behavior of the knee joint with or without menisci. Clin Orthop 149:283–290

Levy IM, Torzilli PA, Warren RF (1982) The effect of medial meniscectomy on anterior, posterior motion on the knee. J Bone Joint Surg 64A:883–888

Mankin HJ, Dorfman H, Lipiello L, Zarins A (1971) Biochemical and metabolic abnormalities in articular cartilage from osteoarthritic human hips. J Bone Joint Surg 53A:523–537
McConaill MA (1932) The function of intraarticular fibrocartilages with special reference to the knee and radio-ulnar joints. J Anat 66:210–227
McGinty JB, Geus LF, Marvin RA (1977) Partial or total meniscectomy: a comparative analysis. J Bone Joint Surg 59A:763–766
Messner K (1994) The concept of a permanent synthetic meniscus prosthesis: a critical discussion after 5 years of experimental investigations using Dacron and Teflon implants. Biomaterials 15:243–250
Milachowski KA, Weismeier K, Erhardt W, Remberger K (1987) Transplantation of the meniscus – an experimental study in sheep. Sportverletz Sportschaden 1:20–24
Milachowski KA, Weismeier K, Wirth CJ, Kohn D (1988) Meniscus transplantation, experimental study, clinical report, arthroscopic findings. In: Müller W, Hackenbruch MH (eds) Surgery and arthoscopy of the knee. Springer, Berlin Heidelberg New York
Milachowski KA, Weismeier K, Wirth CJ (1989) Homologous meniscus transplantation. Int Orthop 13:1–11
Moon MS, Woo YK, Kim YI (1988) Meniscal regeneration and its effects on articular cartilage in rabbit knees. Clin Orthop 227:289–304
Mow VC, Ratcliffe A, Chern KY, Kelly MA (1992) Structure and function relationships of the menisci of the knee. In: Mow VC, Arnoczky SP, Jackson DW (eds) Knee meniscus. Basic and clinical foundations. Raven Press, New York, pp 37–58
Müller W (1994) Menisken und Kniestabilität. Orthopäde 23:93–97
Paletta GA, Manning T, Snell E, Parker R, Bergfeld J (1997) The effect of allograft meniscal replacement on intraarticular contact area and pressures in the human knee – a biomechanical study. Am J Sports Med 25:692–698
Rangger C, Glotzer W, Benedetto KP (1994) Bandinstabilitat nach arthroskopischer medialer Meniskusteilresektion. Unfallchirurg 97:435–437
Seedhom BB, Hargreaves DJ (1979) Transmission of the load in the knee with special reference to the role of the menisci, part II. N Engl J Med 8:220–228
Shelton WR, Dukes AD (1994) Meniscus replacement with bone anchors: a surgical technique. Arthroscopy 10:324–327
Shoemaker SC, Markolf KL (1986) The role of the meniscus in the anterior-posterior stability of the loaded anterior cruciate, deficient knee. J Bone Joint Surg 68A:71–78
Shrive NG, O'Connor JJ, Goodfellow IE (1978) The weight-bearing role of the menisci of the knee. J Bone Joint Surg 56B:381
Smilie JS (1978) Injuries of the knee joint, 5th edn. Livingstone, Edinburgh
Sommerlath K, Gillquist J (1992) The effect of a meniscal prosthesis on knee biomechanics and cartilage. An experimental study in rabbits. Am J Sports Med 20:73–81
Sonne-Holm S, Fledelius J, Ahn NC (1981) Results after meniscectomy in 147 athletes. Acta Orthop Scand 51:303–309
Stone KR, Rodkey WG, Webber RJ, McKinney L, Steadman JR (1990) Future directions: collagen based prostheses for meniscal regeneration. Clin Orthop 252:129–135
Stone KR, Rodkey WG, Webber R, McKinney L, Steadman JR (1992) Meniscal regeneration with copolymeric collagen scaffolds. In vitro and in vivo studies evaluated clinically, histologically, and biochemically. Am J Sports Med 20:104–111
Toyonaga T, Uezaki N, Chikama H (1983) Substitute meniscus of Teflon, net for the knee joint of dogs. Clin Orthop 179:291–297
Van Arkel ERA, De Boer HH (1995) Human meniscal transplantation. J Bone Joint Surg 77B:589–595

Verdonk R, Van Daele P, Claus B, Vandenabeele K, Desmet P, Verbruggen G, Veys EM, Claessens H (1994) Das vitale Meniskustransplantat. Orthopäde 23:153–159

Voloshin AS, Wosk J (1983) Shock absorption of meniscectomised and painful knees: a comparative in vivo study. J Biomed Eng 5:157–161

Walker PS, Erkmann, MJ (1975) The role of the menisci in force transmission across the knee. Clin Orthop 109:184–196

Webber RJ, Zitaglio T, Hough AJ (1986) In vitro cell proliferation and proteoglycan synthesis of rabbit meniscal fibrochondrocytes as a function of age and sex. Arthritis Rheum 29:1010–1016

Wirth CJ, Rodriguez M, Milachowski KA (1988) Meniskusnaht, Meniskusersatz. Thieme Verlag, Stuttgart

Wirth CR (1981) Meniscus repair. Clin Orthop 157:153–160

Zhu W, Chern KY, Mow VC (1994) Anisotropic viscoelastic shear properties of bovine meniscus. Clin Orthop 306:34–45

Zukor DJ, Cameron JC, Brooks PJ, Oakeshott RD, Farine I, Rudan JF, Gross AE (1990) The fate of human meniscal allografts. In: Ewing JW (ed) Articular cartilage and knee joint function: basic science and arthroscopy. Raven Press, New York, pp 147–152

Evaluation of Arthroscopic Techniques and Osteotomies in Gonarthritis

W. Schultz

Introduction

Surgical treatment of gonarthrosis is multifaceted and must thus involve a reference to its limited effectiveness (Hackenbroch 1984). We must differentiate between intra- and extraarticular measures that can be variably combined, depending on the indication. The effectiveness of these interventions should therefore be classified into either *mechanical* or *biological.*

Intraarticular Techniques

Aims, Actions, Indications, Evaluation

The primary focus of intraarticular intervention should be directed at improving the mechanical conditions of the rolling-sliding movement of the knee joint. One effect that cannot be fully calculated is the production of replacement tissue by opening the subchondral cavity. The following sections compare the various techniques.

Debridement or Housecleaning

Cartilage smoothing is a key therapeutic principle in the surgical treatment of arthrosis. The effect involves an improvement in the rolling-sliding mechanism as well as the lavage effect. The latter favorably influences detritus synovialitis. Debridement can be used in all stages of arthrotic degeneration and is particularly effective in the acute phase.

Debridement plus Drilling

Drilling is designed to promote the formation of granulation tissue from the medullary canal. This tissue can differentiate into fibrous cartilage based on the principle of articular movement under minimum stress. Pridie (1951) used drill holes with a diameter of 6 mm; today generally we use a diameter of 2 mm. Advanced arthrosis grades II and III are preferred indications for this technique.

Debridement plus Abrasion Arthroplasty

The original technique was described by Johnson (1986). Reaming goes to a depth of 1–2 mm into the boundary layer; a few years later (1992) he changed his technique. Now the working on the bone surface was more symmetrical and more superficial than before. In this region, vascularization of the cortical bone over the cancellous layer should be good. This facilitates effective repair of the cartilaginous tissue. This technique can only be used in arthrosis grades III and IV, i.e. in largely exposed subchondral bone.

By opening the medullary canal (drilling) or by activating the vessels in the tide mark (abrasion arthroplasty), replacement tissue can be produced and the areas of limited cartilaginous defects filled in with fibrocartilaginous tissue. The disadvantages of this surgical method are that the joint must be kept immobilized longer, the incidence of postoperative bleeding is greater and larger defects are more likely to be filled incompletely.

Clinically, there is no statistical difference between the effects of drilling and abrasion arthroplasty (Schultz 1993). The use of these techniques alone is only justified on joints with correct alignment (Wagner 1976; Klein 1981).

Extraarticular Techniques

Aims, Actions, Indications, Evaluation

The stated aim of corrective osteotomies is to create the most optimal anatomical axial circumstance. Remaining axial defects involve prearthrotic deformities.

Tibial or Supracondylar Femoral Osteotomies

Axial malalignments can be corrected on the tibial side or on the proximal femur. The localization of the osteotomy depends on the alignment of the articular surface in the frontal plane, since the aim is not only to eliminate the axial defect, but also to attempt to align the joint surface horizontally.

Osteotomy is associated with an improvement in the *biomechanical* and the *arthrobiological* situations.

Biomechanics

Some of the beneficial effects of periarticular osteotomies are attributable to an improvement in congruency and a tightening of the ligamentous apparatus, a reduction in pathological pressure points in the joint, an improvement in articular guidance and normalization of cartilage metabolism (Hackenbroch 1982).

Arthrobiological

Other effects of osteotomy are due to the opening of medullary canals, whereby the elevated intramedullary pressure drops and the venous circulation improves (Trueta 1968). The condition of the joint is decisive in establishing the indication for osteotomy. The various types of pain (resting or exercise-related pain) are substantially improved by osteotomy. The pain is perceived as radiating out of the joint, over the joint capsule as well as over the medullary canal of the bone. Closely related interactions between the joint capsule and the subchondral bone have been reported (Willert and Otte 1979). The causes for bone pain, induced by medullary hyperemia and vasodilatation and the associated compression of intraosseous nerve fibers can be correlated with microcirculatory congestion in the sinusoids of the medullary canal observed in arthrosis.

Exercise-stable osteosynthesis is essential for continuous passive motion, which in turn exploits the advantages of the cartilaginous regeneration achieved by these methods (Salter 1986). The disadvantages of osteotomies involve the week-long immobilization of the joint and the potential for nerve lesions, particularly in the case of valgus tibial osteotomies.

Combination of Intra- plus Extraarticular Intervention

Functional disorders of the joint are common in arthrosis and are frequently a manifestation of disturbances of intraarticular structures, neurophysiological dysregulation or even muscular imbalances (Beyer et al. 1990). If clinical examination of a knee joint presenting with axial malalignment reveals symptoms that point to additional damage with locking (meniscus, loose bodies) or extension deficits of the joint due to osteophyte formation in the cruciate ligament fossa or the anterior tibia, we have a clear indication for a combined intervention. By using the combination of intraarticular plus extraarticular intervention (osteotomy), the positive effects of the individual surgical steps become additive. In many cases, joint mobility can be improved immensely by targeted removal of osteophytes, whereby the indication for a joint-preserving intervention can be established at another time. Widespread use of arthroscopic techniques might help lower the risks of surgery.

Results

Published evaluations of the intraarticular measures performed in patients with arthrosis differ, ranging from enthusiastic reports (Rose et al. 1990) through critically positive (Rosenthal et al. 1988; Jennings 1990) to critical and even critically negative appraisals (Grifka 1993; Boe and Hansen 1990). With proper diagnosis, good and satisfactory long-term outcomes have been achieved in a large number of patients with varus or valgus malalignment of the knee joint. Reports on the results achieved with valgus proximal tibial osteotomy are particularly abundant in the literature. The middle-and long-terms results of the osteotomies are shown in Tables 1 and 2.

Table 1. Results of tibial osteotomies

Author	Year	Time of investigation	Number of osteotomies	Results very good\good\satisfactory
Hernigou	1987	5 years	93	90%
Kleinert	1985	6 years	101	75–85%
Rosenkranz	1986	6 years	288	74%
Träger	1989	7 years	34	59%
Wagner	1985	5–9 years	45	82%
Eyb	1988	75 years	74	57%
Bettin	1994	8.5 years	121	80%
Schmitt E	1987	8.8 years	330	79.2%
Coventry/Bowman	1982	10 years	230	62%
Jenny	1985	10 years	106	87%
Fuchs	1994	10.7 years	102	75.81%
Hernigou	1987	11.5 years	93	45%
Heppt	1990	11.9 years	91	52%
Augstburger	1990	13.25 years	62	70%
Schreiber	1986	15 years	78	52%
Wagner	1985	10–17 years	47	81%

Table 2. Results of supracondylar osteotomies

Author	Year	Time of investigation	Number of osteotomies	Results very good\good\satisfactory
Schmitt E	1987	4.2 years	51	70.6%
Wagner	1985	5–9 years	32	81%
Wagner	1985	10–17 years	31	77%
Träger	1989	13 years	25	80%
Legal	1987	14 years	29	75–80%

Combined Procedure

It is possible to combine arthroscopic debridement with osteotomy and either varus or valgus correcting procedures. When the combined procedure is performed at one sitting, the joint debridement is performed first, followed by osteotomy.

Singular reports advocating the combination of extraarticular osteotomy plus intraarticular interventions were published back in the days of arthrotomy (MacIntosh and Welsh 1977; Psczolla and Groeneveld 1984), with no higher risk being shown to result from the additional articular interventions.

But there is no uniform opinion about this. Some of the surgeons cannot do without the intraarticular procedure on principle (Schlegel et al. 1987), while others are looking for clinical symptoms first and operating on the joint when they think it seems to be necessary (Mittelmeier et al. 1990). On the other side there are surgeons doing an initial arthroscopy before osteotomy. Their plans are to establish the diagnosis, and to operate on the meniscus, joint cartilage and osteophytes (Johnson 1986; Naumann et al. 1990).

Therefore, the different handling does not permit a truly critical examination of these procedures. No truly comparative investigations exists. Uniform evaluations and the use of scores is usually missing. Many investigators use subjective factors such as pain, function of the joint and the duration of an ambulatory period free of pain.

In a more recent study (Schultz 1993), the overall clinical outcome was better in patients treated with the combination of osteotomy plus arthroscopy than in patients with osteotomy alone as statistically shown by better mobility – in particular by the better extension of the knee joint – and a longer ambulatory period free of pain (Figs. 1–5).

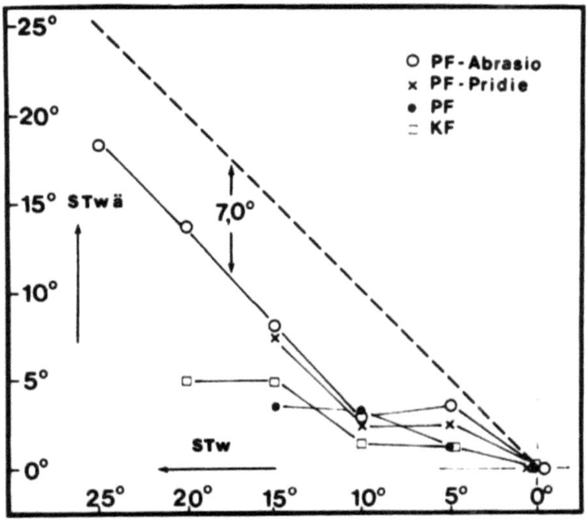

Fig. 1. Change in the extensor angle (*STwä*), plotted as a function of the preoperative status (*STw*) (*preoperative*) of the extension deficit. Abrasion arthroplasty yields very good results for the largest degrees of hypoextension (25–15 °). Even if the extension deficit is not eliminated completely, it can be reduced by up to 7 ° regardless of the preoperative status (*distance to the dotted line*). This convincingly illustrates the statistically validated superiority of the surgical technique with drilling or abrasion arthroplasty. *PF*, plate fixation without joint intervention; *KF*, clamp fixation without joint intervention; *PF – Pridie*, plate fixation with joint intervention (drilling); *PF – Abrasio*, plate fixation with joint intervention (abrasion arthroplasty). Diagram of the pre- and postoperative extension angles and their changes

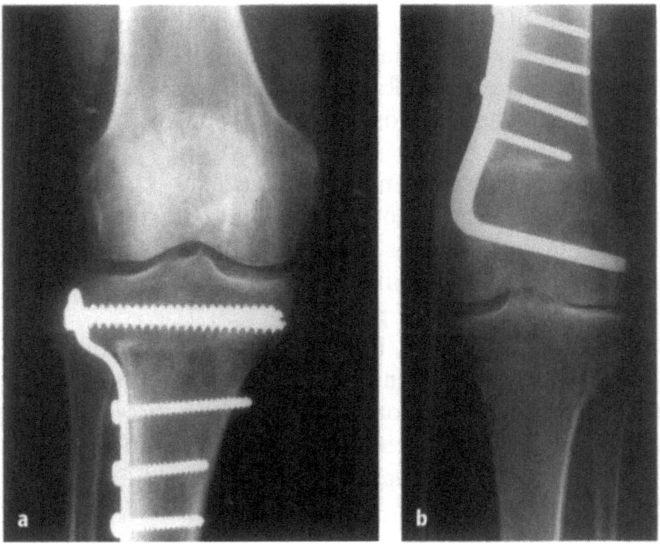

Fig. 2 a, b. Example of the correction of a varus deformity, (**a**) with osteotomy on the proximal part of the tibia and the correction of a valgus deformity, (**b**) with osteotomy at the distal part of the femur with plates

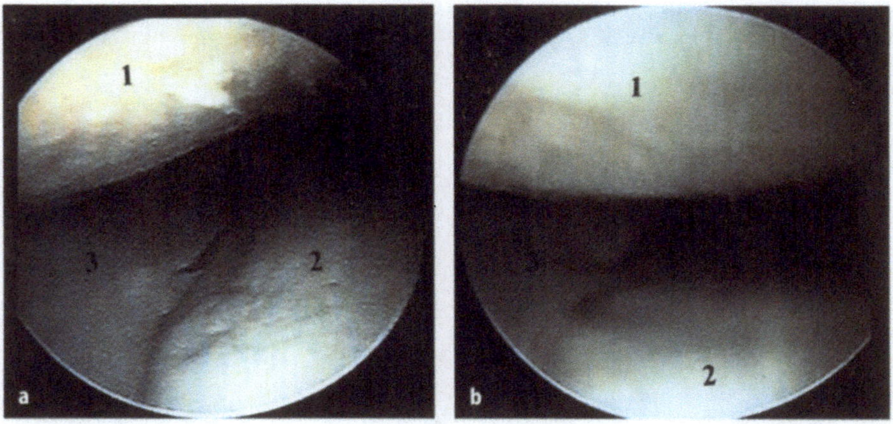

Fig. 3 a, b. Arthroscopic view of the medial joint space **a** before and **b** 14 months after osteotomy without intra – articular surgery. **a** Joint compartment before osteotomy: degenerative changes of the cartilage (grade III and IV) on femurcondyle and the tibia and small changes of the meniscus can be seen. **b** The same joint 14 months after osteotomy: small changes of the cartilage at the tibia and the femurcondyle. The joint appears more smooth and clean than before surgery. (*1*) femurcondyle; (*2*) tibia; (*3*) meniscus

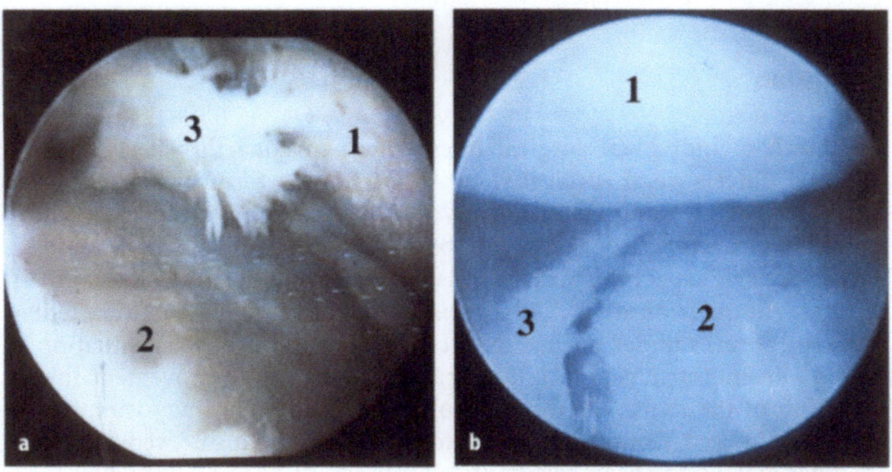

Fig. 4 a, b. Arthroscopic view into a joint, (**a**) before housecleaning (debridement, drilling) with osteotomy and (**b**) 15 months after the combined procedure. **a** Degenerative changes of the cartilage (grade IV) and the meniscus with flaps and tears. **b** Same joint 15 months later: good reparation tissue on the medial condyle and the tibia. The rest of the meniscus appears smooth and solid. (*1*) femurcondyle; (*2*) tibia; (*3*) meniscus

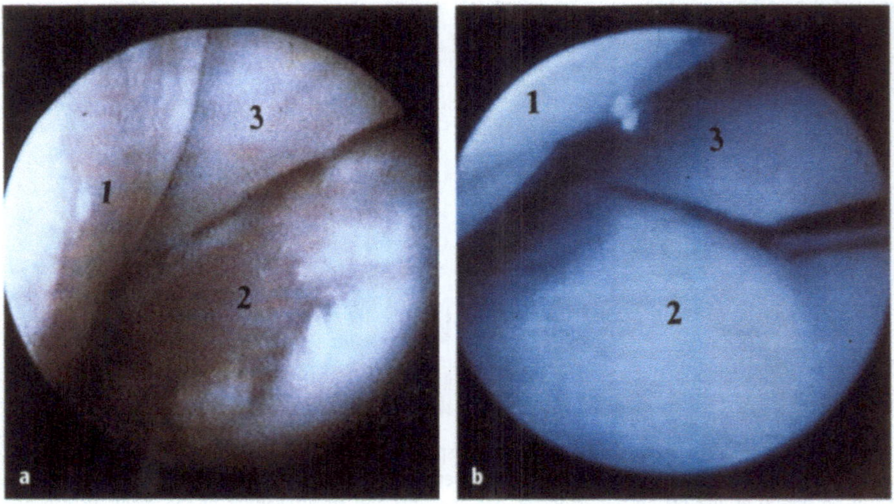

Fig. 5 a, b. Arthroscopic view into a medial compartment with severe degenerative changes (grade IV) of the hyaline cartilage (**a**) before and (**b**) after housecleaning (debridement, abrasion arthroplasty) and osteotomy. **a** The medial joint space before abrasion arthroplasty and osteotomy. **b** The same joint 12 months after osteotomy and abrasion arthroplasty. The femurcondyle and the tibia are covered by good reparation tissue. (*1*) femurcondyle; (*2*) tibia; (*3*) meniscus

Conclusion

The merit of individual surgical intervention in gonarthrosis is difficult to define since several surgical steps are usually performed in concert. In other words, interventions are involved that can improve the mechanical situation, but strictly speaking, cannot actually cure the problem.

One decisive aspect to bear in mind when choosing the route of therapy is certainly the question as to whether *axial malalignment* is present or whether arthrosis prevails under normal axial circumstances. If the axial situation is *normal*, an intraarticular technique can often lead to improvement in the condition of the joint. The duration of this improvement may vary, but is ultimately limited. Contraindications to an intraarticular intervention alone are axial malalignment or instabilities (Wagner 1976; Klein 1981).

The lavage effect of endoscopic housecleaning as a singular procedure can diminish pain, thereby reducing the use of medication, and can considerably prolong the time before further measures are required.

Since no other alternatives are currently available, in patients with arthrosis grades II and III and/or III and IV, and even the course of arthrosis presumably depends on the severity of the chondromalacia (Grifka 1993), it appears sensible to use drilling and abrasion arthroplasty as a last-ditch measure for preserving the joint. The effect of this intervention depends on the size, depth and the diameter of the defect.

In the case of axial malalignment, correction of the axis has immediate priority. For patients with the appropriate indication, the combination of interventions is frequently a blessing because the arthroscopic operation carries a lower risk than arthrotomy and the indication for osteotomy can be broadened to include osteophyte removal in and around the cruciate ligament fossa. When treating injured articular surfaces - and no matter how elegantly - we must realize that we cannot cure the arthrotic condition nor can we stop its progression. However, previous results and experience have shown that these methods can be used to achieve a temporary improvement in subjective symptoms.

In fact, not all arthroscopy possible options should be considered sensible. One should not solely aspire to leave all treated articular surfaces completely flat and smooth, but rather to properly identify any mechanical impediments as such and remove them.

Osteotomy-driven axial correction is also effective in incipient and even advanced arthrosis. The combination of intraarticular intervention plus simultaneous axial realignment depends on the baseline situation of each individual joint at the time the indication for surgery is established. The clinical outcome from these patients is usually much better than in patients with osteotomy alone.

And finally, whenever we plan surgical interventions we should always remember that the damaged cartilage is one major focus of the treatment, but not the only one. In arthrosis, all structures involved in the joint's constitution are altered. This applies to the joint cartilage and the subchondral bone just as much as to the joint capsule and the so called auxiliary structures like the meniscus, ligaments and the musculature.

References

Augstburger F, Knüsel HP, Aebersold P (1990) Langzeitresultate nach valgisierender Tibiakopf-osteotomie bei Varusgonarthrose. Orthop Praxis 2:122–123

Bettin D, Karbowski A, Schilgen M, Saathoff J (1994) Indikation und Therapieerfolg der valgisierenden Tibiakopfosteotomie nach Coventry. Orthop Praxis 3:161–164

Beyer WF, Donner K (1990) Funktionelle Diagnostik von Frühartrosen der Extremitäten. Orthopäde 19:43–49

Blauth W, Döhler JR (1987) Kniegelenksnahe Umstellungsosteotomien. In: Küsswetter W, Krais J (eds) Kniegelenksnahe Osteotomien. Thieme, Stuttgart, pp 10–28

Boe S, Hansen H (1986) Arthroscopic partial meniscectomy in patients aged over 50. J Bone Joint Surg 68B:707–712

Coventry MB (1979) Upper tibial osteotomy for gonarthrosis. The evaluation of the operation in the last eighteen years and long term results. Orthop Clin N Amer 10:191–210

Coventry MB, Bowman PW (1982) Long term results of upper tibial osteotomy for degenerative arthritis of the knee. Acta Orthop Belg 48:139–156

Eyb R, Czurda R, Kristen H (1988) Langzeitergebnisse nach Tibiakopfosteotomie. Orthop Praxis 2:87–93

Fuchs S, Gierse H, Maaz B (1994) Ist die Umstellungsosteotomie am Kniegelenk auch langfristig sinnvoll oder ist heute der Gelenkersatz zeitgemäß? Orthop Praxis 3:165–169

Gariepy R (1964) Genu varum treated by high tibial osteotomy. J Bone Joint Surg 46B:783

Grifka J (1994) Kniegelenksarthrose. Thieme, Stuttgart

Hackenbroch MH (1982) Degenerative Gelenkerkrankungen. In: Handbuch der Orthopädie. Band IV, Allgemeine Orthopädie. Thieme, Stuttgart, pp 1.1–1.56

Hackenbroch MH (1984) Indikationen und Grenzen der nicht achsenkorrigierenden Eingriffe am arthrotisch schwer veränderten Kniegelenk mit Ausnahme der Endoprothetik. Orthop Praxis 11:869–876

Heppt P, Goldmann A, Beyer W, Wirtz P (1990) Indikationen, Risiken und Langzeitergebnisse der valgisierenden Tibiakopf-Pendelosteotomie. Orthop Praxis 2:106–109

Hernigou P, Medevielle D, Debeyre J, Goutallier D (1987) Proximal tibial osteotomy for osteoarthritis with varus deformity. J Bone Jt Surg 69A:332–354

Jennings JE (1990) Arthroscopic surgery in osteoarthritis. In: Glinz W, Kieser CH, Munzinger U (eds) Arthroskopie bei Knorpelschäden und bei Arthrose. Fortschritte in der Arthroskopie, Bd. 6. Enke, Stuttgart, pp 42–44

Jenny K, Jenny H, Morscher E (1985) Indikation, Operationstechnik und Resultate der transcondylären Tibiakopfosteotomie bei Gonarthrose. Orthopäde 14:161–171

Johnson LL (1986) Arthroscopic surgery. Principles and practice. C.V. Mosby, St. Louis Toronto Princetown

Klein W (1981) Indikation zur operativen und konservativen Therapie bei Gonarthrosen mit Achsenabweichungen. Orthop Praxis 3:210–212

Kleinert B, Scheier HJG, Munzinger U, Steiger U (1985) Ergebnisse der Tibiakopf-Osteotomie. Orthopäde 14:154–160

Legal H (1987) Die kniegelenksnahen Osteotomien in der Behandlung der Gonarthrose. Indikation und Ergebnisse. Orthop Praxis 1:53–62

MacIntosh DL, Welsh RP (1977) Joint debridement – a complement to high tibial osteotomy in the treatment of degenerative arthritis of the knee. J Bone Jt Surg 59A:54–61

Mittelmeier H, Schmitt E (1990) Korrekturosteomien im Kniebereich – Indikationen, Grenz- und Kontraindikationen. In: Springorum HW, Katthagen BD (eds) Aktuelle Schwerpunkte der Orthopädie. Thieme, Stuttgart, pp 166–171

Naumann T, Köhler G (1990) Indikationen und Ergebnisse unterschiedlicher knienaher Osteotomieformen bei älteren Patienten mit unilateralen Gonarthrosen – Operationstechnik, Nachbehandlung und Komplikationen. Orthop Praxis 2:118–121

Pridie KH (1959) A method of resurfacing osteoarthritis knee joints. In: Proceedings of the British Orthopaedic Association. J Bone Joint Surg 41B:618–619

Psczolla M, Groeneveld HB (1984) Die Tibiakopfosteotomie mit der AO-Winkelplatte. Orthop Praxis 11:118–121

Rose O, Wuschech H, Kündiger R, Heller G, Pass P (1990) Arthroskopische Operationen am Knorpel des Kniegelenkes. Beitr Orthop Traumatol 37:255–258

Rosenkranz U, Dorn U, Stipicic N (1987) Erfahrungen mit der hohen Tibiakopf-Osteotomie bei Gonarthrose. In: Küsswetter W, Krais J (eds) Kniegelenknahe Osteotomien. Thieme, Stuttgart, pp 121–124

Rosenthal A, Eichhorn J, Nitschke E (1988) Ergebnisse der arthroskopischen Chirurgie bei Gonarthrose. Arthroskopie 1:116–123

Salter RB, Simmonds DF, Malcolm BW, Rumble EJ, McMichael D, Clements ND (1986) The biological effect of continuous passive motion on the healing of full thickness defects in articular cartilage. An experimental investigation in the rabbit. J Bone Jt Surg 62A:1232–1251

Schlegel KF, Müller R (1987) Unsere biologisch und biomechanisch wirksame Schienbeinkopf-Additionsosteotomie mit Gelenktoilette. In: Küsswetter W, Krais J (eds) Kniegelenksnahe Osteotomien. Thieme, Stuttgart, pp 102–109

Schmitt E, Heisel J, Mittelmeier H (1987) Suprakondyläre Umstellungsosteotomien im Kniegelenksbereich. In: Küsswetter W, Krais J (eds) Kniegelenksnahe Osteotomien. Thieme, Stuttgart, pp 34–39

Schmitt O, Schmitt E, Mittelmeier H (1987) Indikation und Technik der kniegelenksnahen Osteotomie bei hemilateraler Gonarthrose mit der Autokompressionsplatte. Orthop Praxis 20:84–89

Schreiber A, Papandreou A, Maygar A, Suter A (1987) 10-Jahresresultate infracondylärer Valgisationsosteotomien bei Gonarthrose. In: Küsswetter W, Krais J (eds) Kniegelenksnahe Osteotomien. Thieme, Stuttgart, pp 49–52

Schultz W (1993) Untersuchungen über die Reparationsmöglichkeiten des chronisch geschädigten Gelenkknorpels am Kniegelenk bei korrigierten Achsenfehlstellungen. Med. Habilitationsschrift, Göttingen

Träger D, Braukmann R, Dybowski W (1989) Kniegelenksnahe Osteotomien-Spätergebnisse. Orthop Praxis 9:585–590

Trueta JM, Harrison HM (1953) The normal vascular anatomy of the femoral head in adult man. J Bone Jt Surg 35B:442–461

Wagner H (1976) Indikation und Technik der Korrekturosteotomie bei der posttraumatischen Kniegelenksarthrose. Unfallheilkunde 128:155–174

Wagner H, Zeiler G, Baur W (1985) Indikation, Technik und Ergebnisse der supra- und infracondylären Korrekturosteotomie bei der Kniegelenksarthrose. Orthopäde 14:172–192

Willert HG, Otte P (1979) Der Gelenkschmerz – Differenzierung arthrogener und osteogener Schmerzkomponenten. Orthop Praxis 1:56–64

Gonarthrosis Treatment According to the "Knee School" Method – A Prospective Randomized Study

E. Broll-Zeitvogel, J. Tyws, A.M. Müller, and J. Grifka

Introduction

Arthrosis of the knee is a significant cause of disability and is of considerable social and medical importance (Molsberger et al. 1993). Arthrosis can be defined as a pathologic joint condition caused by locally degenerative hyaline cartilage and consequent hardening of the subchondral bone (Engel 1994). Clinically it is characterized by pain, muscle imbalance, limited walking, swelling, progressive deformation, and bone destruction.

Continuously increasing exercise pain and start up pain are indicators of gonarthrosis. In addition, what might be called idling pain or rest pain can be observed during inactivity between active phases: constant pain despite rest. These characteristic types of pain combine to render patients progressively immobile.

On the analogy of the "back school" concept (Nentwig et al. 1997), the "knee school" approach (Grifka 1992) educates the patient in anatomy and pathology, and teaches knee-friendly behavior (Figs. 1 and 2). Well-targeted and easy-to-practice exercises help patients to prevent progressive muscular imbalance, as well as to improve mobility and the muscle weakness on their own (Figs. 3 and 4).

Studies into post-arthroscopic therapy of gonarthrosis have shown that knee school practice results in increased insight into the nature of the disorder and recommended behavioral strategy, reducing the feeling of helplessness and depression often found with gonarthrosis patients. This gradually enables them to use their knee joints in normal everyday ways. Even in cases of advanced gonarthrosis, knee school training aims at and brings about reduction of pain and improved knee joint function.

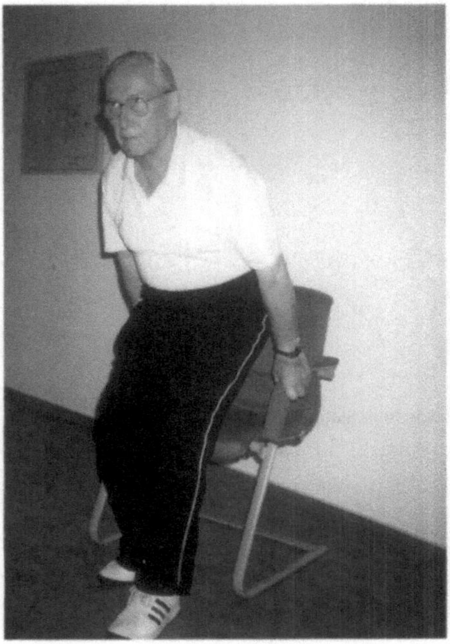

Fig. 1. Knee-friendly standing up from a chair

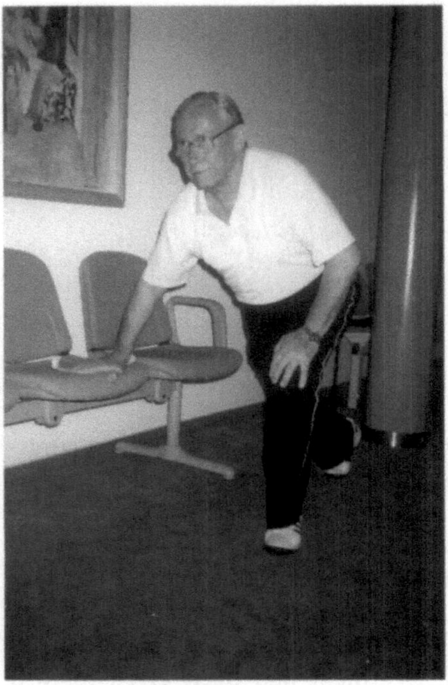

Fig. 2. Knee-friendly standing up and kneeling down

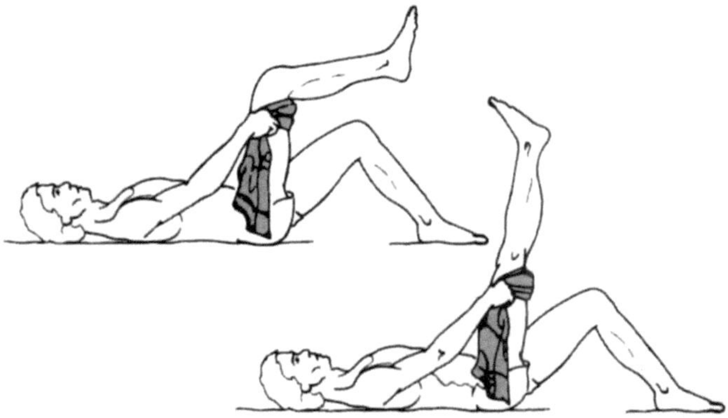

Fig. 3 a, b. Exercise instruction: stretching of knee-flexor musculature (**a**) starting position (**b**) exercise position

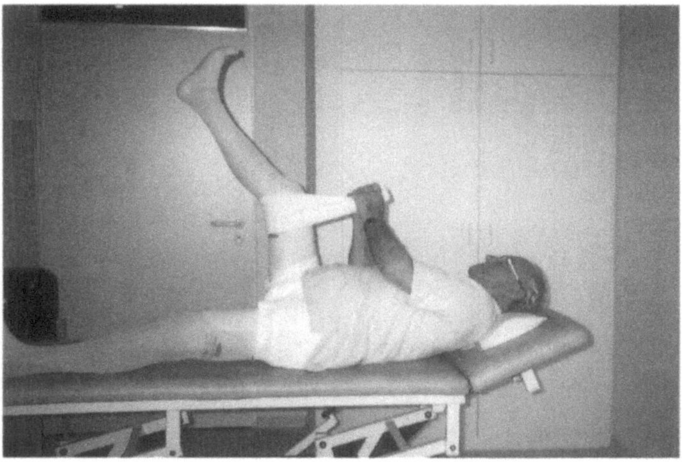

Fig. 4. Exercise performance: stretching of knee-flexor musculature

Subjects and Methods

In total, 98 patients suffering from active gonarthrosis and without surgical intervention were divided into two prospective-randomized groups; a knee school group (KSG) and a control group (CG).

Mean age of the 48 CG patients (29 female 19 male) was 64.2 years as compared to 61.4 years of the 48 KSG patients (31 female, 17 male). Mean duration of pain from initial manifestation to the day of assignment to the study was 32 months (KSG) compared to 34.2 months (CG). Before the start of the study medical treatment had been given to KSG patients for an average 25.1 months and to CG patients for an average 17.2 months (Table 1).

In total, 28 KSG patients (57.1%) and 18 CG patients (36.7%) stated they had reduced quality of life due to knee joint disorders. Both groups were given identical conservative treatment: low frequency therapy, ultrasound treatment, and iontophoresis.

In addition, KSG patients were instructed in knee-friendly behavior according to knee school guidelines (Grifka 1992) – (Table 2). Self-directed exercises to strengthen and stabilize the knee were taught in six consecutive sessions that focussed on pain-free, correct alignment and patterns of movement. No special equipment was required to perform the exercises in the program.

Each of the six knee school training sessions was strictly structured to ensure clarity and compliance, and patients were given illustrated, easy-to-follow instruction booklets. KSG patients were requested to perform the exercise program at home twice a day and to make knee-friendly behavior a habit.

Data were gathered before the start of the study and 3 months after treatment. Patient-related data were obtained by means of five standardized questionnaires covering age, sex, height, weight, profession, duration of pain, intensity of exercise/pain ratio, personal habits such as hygiene, dressing procedures, housework routines, and sports. Additional stan-

Table 1. Patient data

	Knee school group (KSG)	Control-group (CA)
Patients (female/male)	48 (31/17)	48 (29/19)
Mean age (years)	61.4	64.2
Duration of pain (months)	32	34.2
Medical treatment (months)	25.2	17.2

Table 2. Knee school guidelines according to Grifka (1992)

1. Move your body
2. Slim down
3. Relieve your knee joints of excessive physical strain
4. Avoid carrying heavy loads
5. Avoid walking or standing for long periods of time
6. Wear low-heeled shoes
7. Walk on soft soles
8. Avoid extreme bends of your knees
9. Do knee-friendly sports only
10. Exercise the muscles of your legs every day

dardized questions were used to determine the psychological constitution of the patients, their previous knowledge of knee-friendly behavior, and their understanding of potential causes of knee disorders.

Clinical symptoms were recorded using an examination form. In a follow-up interview 3 months later patient compliance was documented, focussing on adherence to knee school guidelines in everyday activities and the frequency of knee school training at home.

Results

Initial Findings

Both groups of patients stated that subjective impairment caused by constant knee pain was their greatest concern. At the beginning of the study there was no significant difference between KSG and CG patients. Both groups of patients had equal intensity of pain, pain while climbing stairs, pain while getting in and/or out of a car etc. (Table 3).

The percentage of patients using special devices like knee bandages or making deliberate efforts at moving as knee-friendly as possible in everyday situations was noted (Table 4). A maximum score of 13 could be achieved for knowledge of the relationship between gonarthrosis, weight, and knee-friendly behavior in everyday conditions. KSG patients scored 9.5 at the onset of the study whereas CG patients scored 10 (Table 4).

Table 3. Experience of pain: statements by the patients

	Initial examination KSG	Initial examination CG	Follow-up KSG	Follow-up CG	Statistical analysis
Subjective impairment through knee pain	47.8%	46.7%	39.2%	41.1%	$p<0.01$ 2-factor analysis
Pain during sudden movements of the knee	78.7	74.5	72.3	87.2	$p<0.05$
Increase of pain while walking on uneven ground	87.5%	93.9%	55.3%	80.0%	
Increase of pain while climbing stairs	62.5%	68.7%	66.7%	85.1%	
Pain while getting in/out of a car	81.1%	63.3%	61.7	60.4%	
Intensity of pain zVAS of pain 0–100	66.2	63.4	52.2	61.3	$p<0.05$

Table 4. Everyday activities/use of special devices

	Initial examination KSG	Initial examination CG	Follow-up KSG	Follow-up CG	Statistical analysis
Use of chairs with armrests	55.1%	51.0%	87.5%	51.0%	$p<0.01$
Doing housework from a sitting position	40.5%	44.4%	76.7%	47.7%	$p<0.01$
Wearing of low-heeled, soft soled shoes	26.5%	32.0%	59.2%	40.8%	
Use of knee bandages	33.3%	36.2%	18.4%	40.4%	$p<0.05$ chi^2-test
Knowledge of knee-friendly behavior and process of arthrosis (max. Score 13)	9.5	10.0	11.3	10.1	

Results of the Follow-up Examination

At 3 months after the initial examination, KSG patients had significantly reduced impairment due to pain ($p<0.01$) and considerably less frequent use of knee bandages. Patients significantly ($p<0.01$) changed their posture doing housework after knee school instruction: KSG patients did their housework more often from a sitting position (Table 4), and they used chairs with armrests to lean on while standing (Fig. 1).

By switching over to the modified pattern of movement recommended, KSG patients were able to reduce pain considerably upon getting in or out of cars ($p<0.01$) (Table 3).

Discussion

Whenever treatment requires active participation by the patient, compliance is a prerequisite for success. As their ailment develops over a long period of time, gonarthrosis patients experience a reduction of mobility and a decrease in social contacts, diminishing the quality of their lives. This is strong motivation to actively improve their situation by whatever means.

The simple, consistent structure of the knee school exercise program makes it easy to grasp. Studies have shown (Loring et al. 1987) that a thorough understanding of a condition is of fundamental importance for the compliance of patients and determines the effect of therapeutic measures. An analysis of 76 studies on the efficiency of patient information revealed that in 61% of the cases, comprehensive and detailed information of the disease resulted in better health and well-being for the patient. The more patients know about their ailment and potential treatment, the greater their compliance (Mayo 1978).

As physiotherapists supervise knee school patients at the beginning of each training session, individual mistakes are noticed and corrected. By regularly doing the exercises of the knee school program on their own patients develop self-discipline. Nonetheless expert support is indispensable.

Weseloh et al. (1990) were able to show that the long-term nature of their ailment is a key factor in compliance of the gonarthrosis patient. They examined 420 people with a high risk of arthrosis who had not yet developed it: 50% of those taking part in the study didn't continue their preventive exercise program because of a lack of motivation or time.

Restoring well-balanced, strong thigh muscles is important to prevent atrophy of vastus medialis and consequent muscular imbalance. Being the key muscle of the knee joint, the vastus medialis atrophies quickly when inactive and easily loses functional activity (Börnert 1991; Dippold 1981). This type of atrophy can be defined as a segmental, spinal motor regulatory disorder, representing a neuropathic myogenous tissue syndrome with volumetric and isometric type-II fiber atrophy (Ziegan and Dippold 1985). It causes inadequate control and misplaced load of the knee joint, constant overload of its capsule-ligament structure and effusions into the joint. There is cartilage-wear due to excessive, permanent strain (Börnert 1991; Dippold 1981).

Dippold (1981) proved that long and intensive tensing up of the muscles has a positive effect on type-II fibers. Knee school exercises increase maximum strength and – in the long run – improve inter- and intramuscular coordination, which patients find beneficial in everyday situations (Grifka et al. 1993).

The fact that motivation has to be considered a key element of successful training was shown by Börnert (1991) and Dippold (1981) who found that supervised isometric muscle training did not yield results unless the patients were determined to make the greatest possible effort.

Previous studies by Grifka et al. (1993) proved positive effects of knee school practice after arthroscopic knee surgery. The present study shows considerable improvement of symptoms after strictly conservative treatment.

Conclusion

This study has proved that the combination of muscle strengthening knee school exercises geared to the needs of gonarthrosis patients and instruction on knee-friendly behavior in everyday situations results in considerable alleviation of pain and improved function of the knee joint.

Due to reduced pain and improved mobility, patients showed more positive psychological states and reported a general increase in the quality of life. This in turn makes social re-integration easier and therefore meets the needs of elderly patients in particular.

References

Börnert K (1991) Trainingseffekte am neuromuskulären System „Kniegelenk". Dtsch Z Sportmed 42:96–102

Dippold A (1981) Die Objektivierung von Muskelfunktionsstörungen bei Arthrose am Modell des Kniegelenks. Beitr Orthop Traumatol 28:109–115

Engel JM (1994) Schmerztherapie der Arthrose. Internist 35:41–48

Grifka J (1992) Die Knieschule. Rowolth, Reinbek

Grifka J, Kraushaar K, Windemuth D (1993) Die Knieschule – Übungsprogramm und Verhaltensmaßnahmen im Alltag. Med Orth Tech 113:86–92

Loring K, Konkol L, Gonzales V (1987) Arthritis patient education: a review of the literature. Patient Education and Counselling 10:207–252

Mayo NE (1978) Patient compliance: practical implications for physical therapists. Phys Ther 58:1083–1090

Molsberger A, Lorek M, Jensen KU (1993) Die Korrelation von Röntgenbefund, Schmerzintensität und subjektiv empfundener Beeinträchtigung bei Gonarthrose. Z Orthop 2:159–163

Nentwig C, Krämer J, Ullrich CH (1997) Rückenschule: Verhaltenstraining zur Prävention und Rehabilitation degenerativer Wirbelsäulenerkrankungen. Enke, Stuttgart

Weseloh G, Mühlbayer P, Hofmann G (1990) Akzeptanz langfristiger krankengymnastischer Übungsprogramme zur Prävention von Arthroseprozessen in Hüft- und Kniegelenken. Akt Rheumatol 15:225–232

Ziergan J, Dippold A (1985) Charakteristische morphologische Veränderungen des M. vastus medialis bei Gonarthrose. Beitr Orthop Traumatol 32:26–29

Knee School: Practical Management in Rehabilitation

J. Kirmair

Introduction

Knee problems have become illnesses of civilization because of loss of use or overuse of functional chains, lack of movement, too much sitting, obesity, and lack of physical training.

In addition to back and neck/shoulder problems, the knee is a common and frequent reason for consulting a doctor for treatment and/or a prescription for sick-leave from work. Knee problems result in dysfunction of the legs, with side effects in somatic, psychological, professional, recreational and social domains. With back pain, experience has shown that, besides the therapeutic program the patient should be educated about prevention in order to diminish or stop an increase in problems. Similar results apply to knee problems. It may be possible to relieve knee problems by decreasing risk patterns of behavior.

Like the back school for problems of the vertebral column, Joachim Grifka developed the idea of a knee school. It has proved its effectiveness according to reports in literature.

We introduced our knee school as a supplementary treatment during rehabilitation in our orthopaedic clinic.

Principles

The knee school consists of modification of behavior and a physiotherapeutic program to stretch the shortened soft tissues and strengthen the muscles.

The aims of rehabilitation in modifying behavior are as follows:
- Reducing overload of the knee joint
- Developing a knee-protective behavior
- Learning new patterns of movement
- Improving movement coordination
- Joint protection in everyday life situations
- Achieving greater activity despite the illness.

Behavior modification involves education about everyday situations that overload the knee joint and therefore should be avoided (Fig. 1), instruction in knee-protective behavior and practical training in order to learn and improve the new pattern of movement. Practical applications are demonstrated and discussed.

The patient must have the capacity to receive and act upon the new information, be willing to change his behavior, learn the new patterns of movement and apply them in everyday life at home and work.

For the behavior modification, it is most effective to teach in small groups in order to benefit from the model learning effect - as has proved effective in back schools (Fig. 2). The group spreads a positive dynamism among its members. Knee school is in part a teaching of an attitude; to be more conscious of and more responsible for one's own health by changing behavior while standing, moving, bending, carrying and doing sports. At all times one should pay attention to the principles of joint protection. Finally, the affected person should be able to regain enough competence to help himself and to adapt his living conditions accordingly.

The principles of the knee school are summed up in ten rules, as follows:

1. Maintain movement
2. Decrease weight
3. Unload the knee joint
4. Avoid lifting or carrying heavy objects
5. Avoid long periods of standing or walking

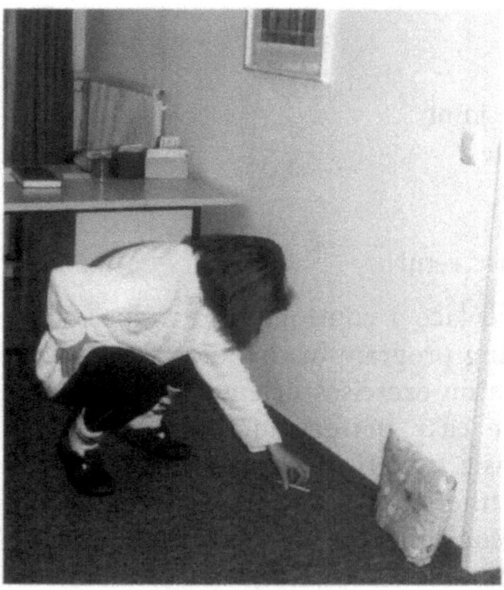

Fig. 1. Example of a bad pattern of movement – overcharging the knee joints while lifting

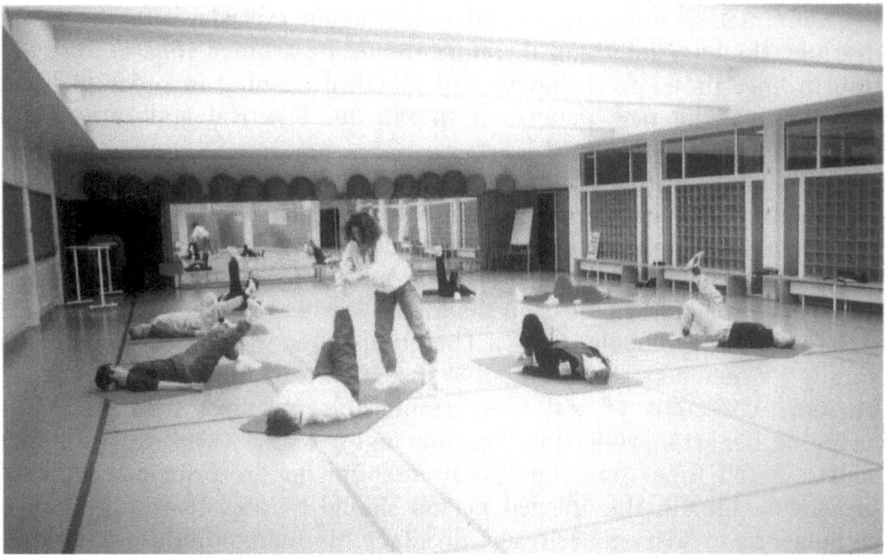

Fig. 2. The knee school group in action. The therapist can supervise and instruct each patient

6. Wear shoes with low heels
7. Wear shoes with yielding soles
8. Avoid extreme bending of the knee
9. Do sports that are suitable for your knee
10. Train leg muscles daily.

In a knee school program, the training in practice by physiotherapy is as important as behavior modification. The aims of rehabilitation in physiotherapy are as follows:

1. Strengthening of muscles
2. Stable muscular movement of knee joint
3. Lengthening of shortened soft tissues
4. Reduction of muscular inequalities
5. Improving joint metabolism
6. Improving the venous and lymphatic return.

It is not the aim of knee school to replace a controlled individual physiotherapy program. The special training program of the knee school consists of muscular contraction and motion exercises orientated in the simple knee axes. The advantage is the easy performance, the exact frequency, the good response of the phasic type II fibers by long and intensive contraction of the muscles and therefore improvement of maximal force and inter- and intramuscular coordination. The sequence of contraction exercises (in order to stabilize the knee joint), and the number and frequency of repetitions, represents training for force-endurance according to Harre (1982).

Management and Organization

We organized the knee school in our rehabilitation center as follows: Patients who had undergone surgery just before coming to us or who had restrictions in bending or loading their knee joints imposed by the surgeon, were treated only by physiotherapy. The rest of the patients with knee problems took part in the knee school as a supplementary treatment. During the first week of the patient's stay we offered four sessions of instructions/exercises:

1. At first we offered 30–45 min of theoretical information that included the basic mechanism of the knee, explanation of the function of the articular components, and principles of joint metabolism. We gave further explanations of the knee school rules, and motivated patients for the following three practical sessions.
2. Afterwards we gave three sessions (30 min each) of practical instructions with repetition of the corresponding knee school rules and demonstration in practice. Devices used are mat, stool, roll and towel. The training program consists of motion exercises and isometric muscular contractions as well as patterns of movement in a diagonal plane.

We integrate a training program for lengthening the muscular tendinous structures:

- First practical unit consists of exercises on the stool (Figs. 3 and 4).
- Second practical unit consists of exercises in the supine position.
- Third practical unit consists of exercises in the prone (Figs. 5 and 6) and side positions.

After attending the knee school – after the first week of the patient's stay in the clinic – the patients took part in group physiotherapy. Patients with knee problems were assembled in groups doing kinesiotherapy on the ground and in the pool.

In a clinic for rehabilitation there are other means of physical therapy for treatment of knee problems, which should be used as required. Other concurrent problems may also be present and need to be treated.

Study Design

In 1995, our clinic for orthopedic rehabilitation carried out a prospective randomized study with a total of 120 patients, distributed into a knee

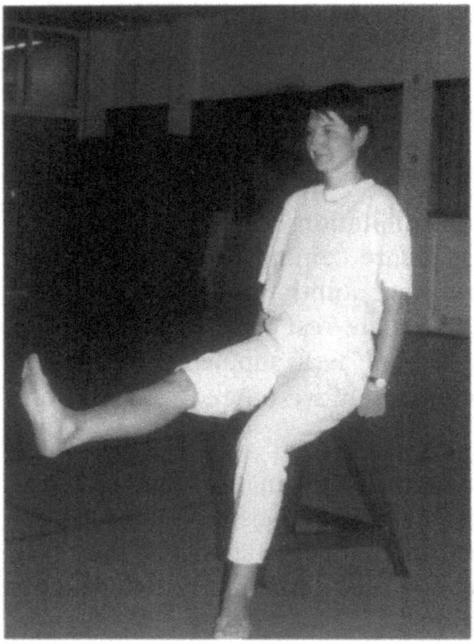

Fig. 3. Example for an exercise on the stool. Isometric muscular contraction .ll as movement in a diagonal plane

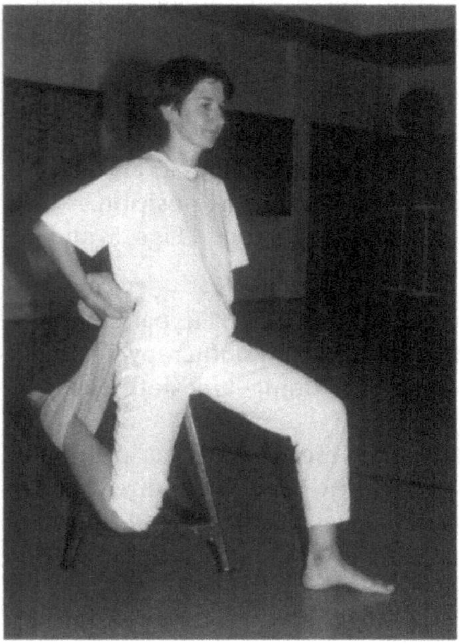

Fig. 4. Example of an exercise on the stool. Lengthening the muscular tendinous structures

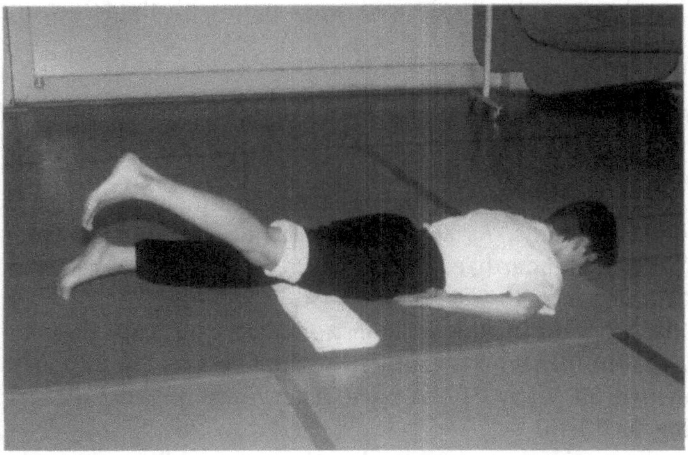

Fig. 5. Example of an exercise in the prone position. Muscular contractions and motion exercises orientated in the simple knee axes

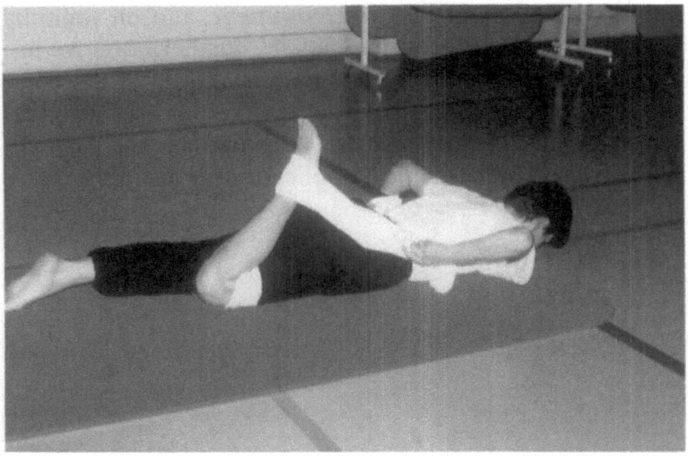

Fig. 6. Example of an exercise in the prone position. Lengthening the muscular tendinous structures

school group and a control group (with proportional distribution of age and sex). All patients in the study were examined and questioned by the same investigator. This was carried out before (first examination) and after attending (second examination) the knee school and before discharge (third examination). All 120 patients were followed without drop-outs. We examined the changing parameters during the patient's stay (4 weeks) for all patients, and comparing the knee school with the control group. We made a two-factor comparing analysis with repeating of one factor.

Criteria for taking part in this study were knee pain with the following diagnoses:

- Gonarthritis
- Knee ligament instability
- Anterior knee pain.

On average the patients had undergone medical treatment because of knee problems for 104 months. As almost all patients also suffered from back pain, we made a standardized therapeutic program for the knee joint and the vertebral column.

The investigation program included a questionnaire, physical examination, and estimation of behavior in practical application. In 87 cases (72.5%) we performed an X-ray of the knee. The grade of arthritis was classified according to Wirth.

We questioned the patients regarding duration of inability to work, their occupation, problems in getting in or out of a car, how long they had been driving a car. At check-ups during the treatment stage, we asked for the walking range and the duration of sitting. The improvement in the subjective knee pains at rest, on movement, and on walking upstairs was marked on a visual scale by the patient. Furthermore, we inquired, by questionnaire, about the theoretical understanding of the condition by the patient. The patient's behavior was assessed in everyday situations - sitting down (Fig. 7), sitting (Fig. 8), kneeling (Figs. 9 and 10) and going upstairs (Fig. 11). Their practical application in avoiding inap-

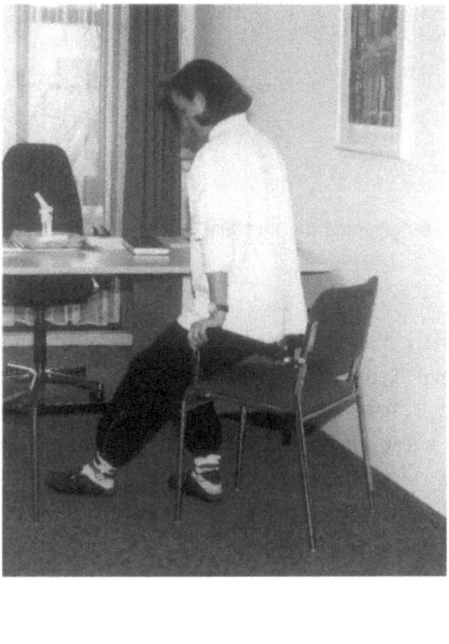

Fig. 7. Example of a good pattern of movement while sitting down

propriate knee joint movements and making better knee movements was estimated. During the second and third examinations we asked the patient's opinion about the effectiveness of the therapy in improving their knee problems.

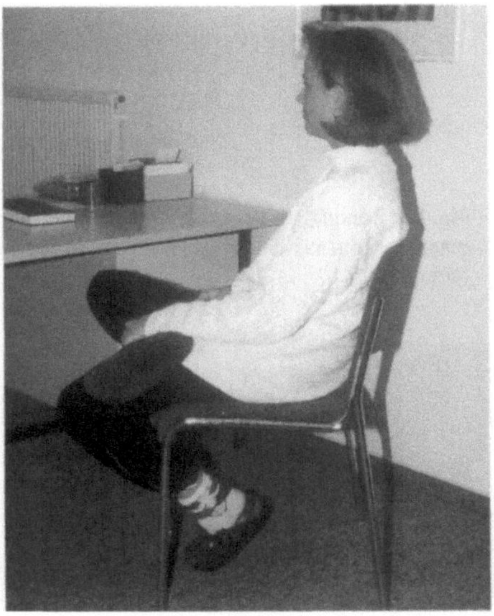

Fig. 8. Example of a bad position while sitting overburdening the knee joints

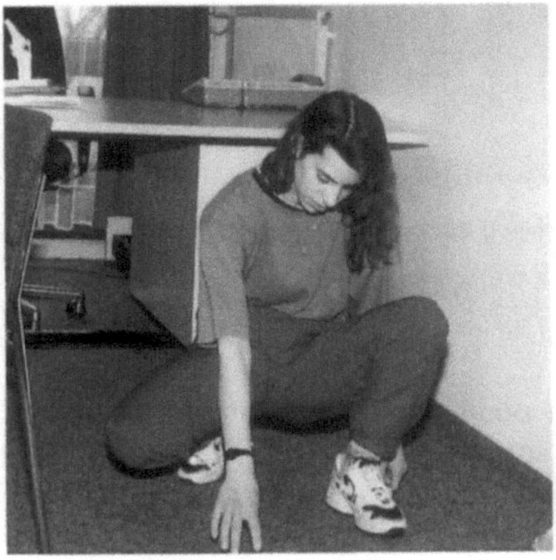

Fig. 9. Example of a bad pattern of movement overcharging the knee joints while kneeling (see Fig. 10)

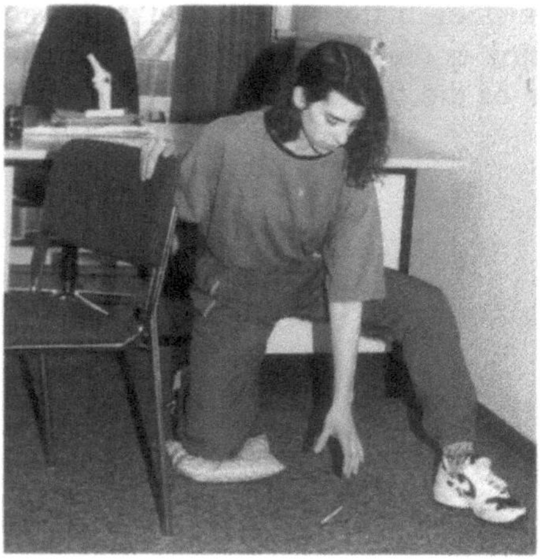

Fig. 10. Example of a good pattern of movement. Performance of the same task as in Fig. 9 (lifting)

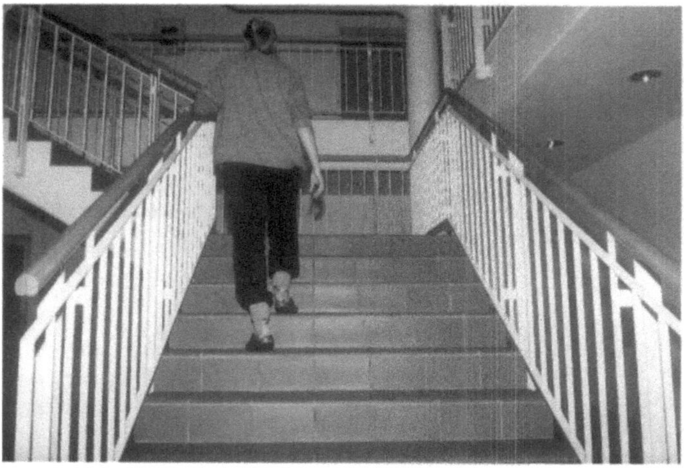

Fig. 11. Example of a good pattern of movement while going upstairs by using the banisters

Results

The parameters of pain at rest, pain on motion, duration in the sitting position, behavior assessment of the sitting position and the patient's assessment of the effectiveness of the knee therapy were not statistically significantly different either during the 4-week period of the patient's stay, or between the knee school group and control group.

For all patients there was a highly statistically significant improvement in knee pain while going upstairs and a statistically significant improvement of the walking range and the objective behavior assessment while going upstairs.

The objective behavior assessment while sitting down and kneeling showed a statistically significant improvement for all patients. In addition there was a statistically significant difference between the knee school group and control group for the kneeling, and the sitting down.

In questioning understanding of the theory and its practical application there was a statistically highly significant improvement for all patients as well as a statistically significant difference between the knee school group and the control group before discharge from our clinic.

Conclusions

Our knee school study showed a statistically significant improvement concerning the theoretical understanding of knee problems and practical application of objective behavior assessment of the motion patterns sitting down and kneeling. These are complex motion patterns that need, for the most part, new instructions and training in practice so they can be memorized.

During the 4-week stay in our rehabilitation center, the study showed a statistically highly significant improvement regarding the knee pain while going upstairs and the theoretical understanding, a statistically significant improvement regarding the objective behavior assessment of the motion patterns sitting down, kneeling and going upstairs as well as the walking range in all our patients. This indicates we achieved success in rehabilitation in all patients and shows the quality and acceptance of our therapeutic program.

We see indications for knee school in cases of gonarthritis, knee ligamentary instability and anterior knee pain. The knee school helps conservative treatment, postoperative treatment and in prevention of deterioration.

The particular advantages of knee school are the instruction in small groups. The group dynamics promote patient motivation and patients benefit from the effect of model learning (behavior therapy).

An instruction program in four sessions has proved necessary in order to repeat the information, and deepen the knowledge about knee. Overall, the patient's understanding about knee problems is increased. In particular they are taught to avoid inappropriate knee joint movements and otherwise make better knee movements in daily situations (Fig. 12) at home and at work.

We emphasize the advantage of a longer period of treatment in a clinic for rehabilitation: by being protected from stressful situations at home and at work the patient can concentrate and focus on his/her own recovery.

They can adopt healthier ways of living and a more favorable behavior, practicing new patterns of movement in small groups and reflecting on

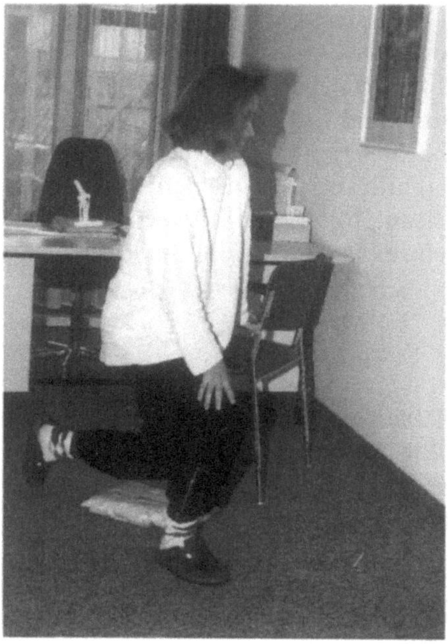

Fig. 12. Example for a good pattern of movement while kneeling down

these new experiences. In the clinic, the patient meets many people who can help in problem solving - doctors, therapists, psychologists, social workers and other patients. Together they form the rehabilitation team - and their cooperation is important and decisive for the patient's motivation for recovery.

Further Reading

Brehm W (1987) Kompetent altern mit Sport. Z Gerontol 20:336-344
Broll-Zeitvogel E, Tyws J, Grifka J, Müller AM (1999) Die Knieschule in der postoperativen Therapie der Gonarthrose - Prospektiv randomisierte Studie. Arthroskopie (in press)
Fliegel S, Groeger WM, Künzel R, Schulte D, Sorgatz H (1981) Verhaltenstherapeutische Standardmethoden. Urban & Schwarzenberg, Munich
Grifka J (1992) Die Knieschule - Hilfe bei Kniebeschwerden. Rowohlt, Reinbek
Grifka J, Kraushaar K, Windemuth D (1993) Die Knieschule - Übungsprogramm und Verhaltensmaßnahmen im Alltag. Med Orth Tech 113:86-92
Harre D (1982) Trainingslehre. Sportverlag, Berlin
Hermann JM, Gaus E (1981) Die klinische Bedeutung der Compliance. Schweiz Med Wschr 111:1998-2005
Heuwinkel D (1990) Sport für Ältere in einer sportaktiven alternden Gesellschaft. Z Gerontol 23:23-33
Jokl P, Stull PA, Lynch J, Vaughan V (1989) Independent home versus supervised rehabilitation following arthroscopic knee surgery - a prospective randomized trial. Arthroscopy 5:298-305

Kopp P (1993) Bewegungstherapeutische Nachbehandlung nach arthroskopischer Therapie der Gonarthrose. Arthroskopie 6:212–217
Kunz HR, Schneider W, Spring H, Tritschler T, Inauen EU (1990) Krafttraining. Thieme, Stuttgart
Nentwig CG, Krämer J, Ullrich CH (1990) Die Rückenschule. Enke, Stuttgart
Rippey RM, Bill D, Abeles M, Day J, Downing DS, Pfeifer CA, Thal SE, Wetstone SL (1987) Computer-based patient education for older persons with osteoarthritis. Arthritis Rheum 30:932–935
Schreiner CH, Grifka J, Windemuth D (1994) Die Knieschule bei Gonarthrose. Orthop Praxis 4:214–217
Ullrich CH, Nentwig CG, Windemuth D (1990) "Knieschule" bei Gonarthrosen. Therapiewoche 40:453–455
Windemuth D, Grifka J, Kirmair J. Knieschule. In: Nentwig CG, Neumann W, Krämer J (eds) Psychologie in der Orthopädie. Hogrefe, Göttingen (in press)

Psychologic Aspects of Training Therapy

D. Windemuth

Introduction

Numerous psychological concepts and theories are of importance for training therapy. For example basic psychologists focus on the measurement of motivation as well as on cognitive or emotional aspects in sports or therapy. In contrast, for social psychologists the dynamic of a group is the most important for training therapy. They also check the significance of the opinion leaders in a team or a group of patients and use them to obtain the most benefit. The task of an educational psychologist is to design the best way to learn. The most important field of applied psychology in training therapy is clinical psychology. Therapy of patients with chronic pain or psychosomatic diseases is only one of their tasks that has achieved recognition in recent years.

The concept of *health locus of control* from the psychology of personality is currently topical.

The Concept of Health Locus of Control

The concept of *locus of control* is currently one of the most investigated areas in psychology. The concept makes it possible to state the expectations or convictions of a person and the way to achieve improvement. People can expect to improve health as a consequence of their own behavior. Alternatively, they may believe that the achievement is not influenceable. Along such a continuum, expectancies can be arranged as either internal or external. Rotter (1966), who introduced this concept in the frame of his social learning theory (1954), calls the poles of the continuum internal or external locus of control.

“When a reinforcement is perceived by the subject as following some action of his own but not being entirely contingent upon his action, then, in our culture, it is typically perceived as the result of luck, chance, fate, as under control of powerful others, or as unpredictable [...] when the event is interpreted in this way by an individual, we have labeled this a belief in *external control.* If the person perceives that the event is contingent upon his own behavior or his own relatively permanent characteristics, we have termed this a belief in *internal control*" (p1).

In the 1970s the external beliefs theory became further differentiated. Following Levenson (1972), it was divided into a social-externality and a chance-externality. Social-externality expresses the conviction that changes are influenced by powerful other persons (p-externality); chance (or c-) externality defines the belief that they are the result of luck or fate. The three dimensions, internality, c- and p-externality are independent of each other. The scores are distributed in a normal way on every dimension. Thus, someone can believe in achieving a target through his own behavior (high internality) but that in addition the help of powerful others is necessary. Independent of this, the role of luck in the change can perceived as large or small.

The behavior of a person can be predicted with the help of this locus of control. Numerous studies proved that an internal locus of control predicts the execution of a behavior for the acquisition of an attractive target, while during high c-externality the behavior is not executed. In case of high p-external belief people would prefer action that fulfills the demands of another important person.

Such global locus of control can predict behavior in many areas of life but this prediction is quite inaccurate. That is why Rotter (1975) required assessment of locus of control specifically for those situations in which behavior has to be predicted. It is possible that a person has an internal locus of control in one area of life, yet in another a strongly c-external belief (e.g. if a person believes he can influence his state of health, but for vocational success he needs good relations with a superior). In response to Rotter's demand, a set of possibilities was developed to measure locus of control in specific areas. One of these areas was health and illness, which is based on Wallston et al. (1976).

Health locus of control is the belief of a person whereby his health is controlled (e.g. Wallston et al. 1978). A person can be convinced that he has control of his health status (internality) or that he does not have any control because of powerful other persons (p-externality) or general lack of control (c-externality). This health locus of control permits prediction of health-related behavior to a considerable degree. The relevance for the success of training therapy is obvious, because self-directed behavior is necessary to achieve success.

In 1976, the first questionnaires for assessing health locus of control were developed (Wallston et al. 1976). This still quite simple scale was refined and differentiated in later years (Wallston et al. 1978). In the late 1980s in Germany scales were developed by Lohaus and Schmitt (1988), Böhlen (1988) Ferring and Filipp (1989) and Mrazek (1989). Later they became further specialized, e.g. particularly for diabetic patients (Kohlman et al. 1993). Beside questionnaires, other procedures for the assessment of locus of control were developed (e.g. interviews); but they did not achieve wide use.

In the 1980s, assessment of locus of control played an increasing role in the field of behavioral medicine. The research reaches from the investigation of connections, e.g. between locus of control and preventive health behavior, up to attempts to predict the success of a therapy or operation by locus of control. After a more general overview, we will discuss particularly the area of orthopaedics.

Connections Between Locus of Control and Convalescence

The following will deal with possibilities of operationalization the convalescence briefly. The psychological beginnings for the prediction of the convalescence do not refer yet to locus of control. Later the development of practice-relevant research presented locus of control as a predictor for organic convalescence. The relevance for training therapy becomes important by that variable.

Possibilities to Operationalize the Construct Convalescence

The term *convalescence* has been reported in different ways. The simplest measure for convalescence is the number of days a patient stays in a hospital (e.g. after an operation). This is an easy but not a valid way to measure convalescence because it does not sufficiently reflect the extent of subjective condition or organic recovery. Further factors, e.g. the number of patients in the hospital, are likewise important factors of influence on this measure. Because the judgement (e.g. of physicians) over the state of health of a patient correlates poorly with the patient's well-being, the interpretation of this measure requires caution. Therefore, it is advisable to determine the recovery of patients multifactorially in the sense of the World Health Organization Ottawa Charter (1986). This would include the subjective well-being of the patient. The specification of the criteria that measures convalescence is indispensable. Such a global kind of operationalization is introduced later.

First Empirical Findings of Predicting Convalescence by Psychological Variables

Research on prediction of convalescence refers predominantly to the recovery status after an operation. Frequently, prediction of the result of an operation by medical rather than psychosocial variables was tried. A sample of patients following back surgery was selected in many studies. Reasons for the selection of this sample are the frequently unsatisfactory results of the operation (Hirsch 1965; Schwetschenau et al. 1976) and the difficulty in prediction of the results from a medical point of view alone (Roberts et al. 1984). A good prediction of the reduction of pain intensity after traditional disc surgery was made successfully by medical variables (Weir 1979).

Numerous studies exist in which multidimensional personality inventories such as the Minnesota Multiphasic Personality Inventory (MMPI) are used to predict the success of an operation. The results are relatively uniform. Patients with minimal improvement reach increased values on the subscales hysterias and hypochondrias (Wiltse and Rocchio 1975; Oostdam and Duivenvoorden 1983) or additionally on the subscale depression. Comparable results were supplied by some (Valach et al. 1988) but not others (Waring et al. 1976). In these studies, psychological variables correctly account for the classification of 87% of the operated patients. These findings are problematic in that no conclusion can be reached about the cause and the effect (increased values on the MMPI subscales hysterias, hypochondrias and depression can be, but do not have to be, the cause of a surgery failure). Comparable scale profiles are also shown by patients with minimal organic diagnosis for disc complaints (Hanvik 1951; Calsynet al. 1976) or patients with a very long duration of complaint before surgery (Hasenbrink and Ahrens 1987; Sternbach et al. 1973) or for patients with chronic pain (Merskey and Boyd 1978).

Nevertheless, with careful interpretation these results permit relevant conclusions for clinical practice, as discussed by Wiltse and Rocchio (1975). From the results they derive conservative indications for surgery. With objective medical results, which justify surgery, an operation should be performed independently of the results of the psychological test. If the patient shows favorable test results, pronounced pain symptoms, but minimal objective medical results, a surgery is to be endorsed, since symptom reduction after surgery is probable. With unfavorable MMPI results, high pain intensity and minimal objective results, an operation should be avoided, since a symptom reduction is improbable.

Thus, the dilemma of this research consists in the fact that it does not permit conclusions in a causal way, because the scale profile of the MMPI does not permit a prediction of the relevant behavior. It is more effective to measure parameters, such as health locus of control, which enable a direct prediction of behavior. In the ideal case this variable can predict the behavior that has influence on the convalescence. A causality can be proven only conditionally, but it can be substantiated by plausibility.

Locus of Control as Predictor of Organic Convalescence

One of the first studies into the connection between health-referred cognition and convalescence was accomplished by Rogner et al. (1987). They showed that only 17% of the variance in the recovery of patients can be explained by the severity level of the injury. This variance could be increased to 48% by inclusion of different psychological variables. An internal locus of control was proved to be favorable for the convalescence. However, the convalescence was defined as the period spent in the hospital and by the judgement of the physician.

Later studies were able to confirm the connection for different groups of patients, although the criterion variables were not always directly related to convalescence. For example Schulze et al. (1988) found a connection between locus of control and post-surgical psychological symptoms in women after hysterectomy; Schumacher et al. (1987) found the connection for patients after extracorporal treatment of nephritic stones; Partridge and Johnston (1989) for patients after a traumatic brain injury and patients with a fracture of the wrist, and Windemuth et al. (1991) for surgical patients after rupture of a ligament of a knee joint. Usually, on any given criteria, a favorable effect can be shown for patients with high internality and an unfavorable effect for patients with high c-externality.

Studies in Samples of Orthopaedic Patients

For orthopaedic patients the prediction of health status by health locus of control offers itself as a useful tool, because a large number of diseases can be influenced by the patients through their own behavior. Because of this, training therapies such as knee schools (Grifka 1992), back schools (Nentwig et al. 1997) and shoulder schools (Windemuth and Ullrich 1997) have been established. This therapeutically important behavior should be predictable by health locus of control and this behavior should control the convalescence. Other areas of convalescence, which cannot be affected directly by own behavior, should not be predictable.

Two studies are presented briefly (further details can be found in Windemuth 1991). These studies clarify the enormous importance of locus of control for the success of training therapy. Finally, we will discuss the practical possibilities of considering this variable in the planning and organization of training therapy.

Study I: Locus of Control and the Success of a Shoulder and a Knee School

The sample of the first study consists of $n=54$ patients with chronic shoulder complaints and of $n=148$ patients with chronic knee complaints. The diagnosis for the shoulder patients is impingement syndrome I or II (classification according to Neer 1983), i.e. exclusion of patients with indications for a surgery. Complaints were due to impingement of the supraspinatus tendon. In addition to the conservative medical treatment, about half of the patients participated in a shoulder school (shoulder schools in general: Hedtmann and Fett 1988). The diagnosis of the knee patients was gonarthrosis, and chondromalacia patellae.

The shoulder and the knee schools are behavior training programs, which inform patients in groups about the anatomy of the shoulder or knee, the pathological changes associated with the symptoms and the possibilities of contributing to the convalescence by purposeful gymnastic exercises. At the same time patients are instructed in the technique of systematic self-monitoring. Four to five weeks later a further session was given with the goal of deepening the technique of self-monitoring and of controlling the correct execution of the exercises.

The extent of convalescence of the shoulder was evaluated with the help of a modified version of the Constant scale (Constant and Murley 1987) on five occasions: before the start of treatment as well as 1, 2, 4 and 6 weeks after (Fig. 1). The following measures were used: pain (pain on movement and rest defined by the patients and also classified by the physician with analgesic use as a guideline); the extent of functional impairment because of pain; muscular strength (when carrying weights keeping the arms hanging, as well as with different movements of the

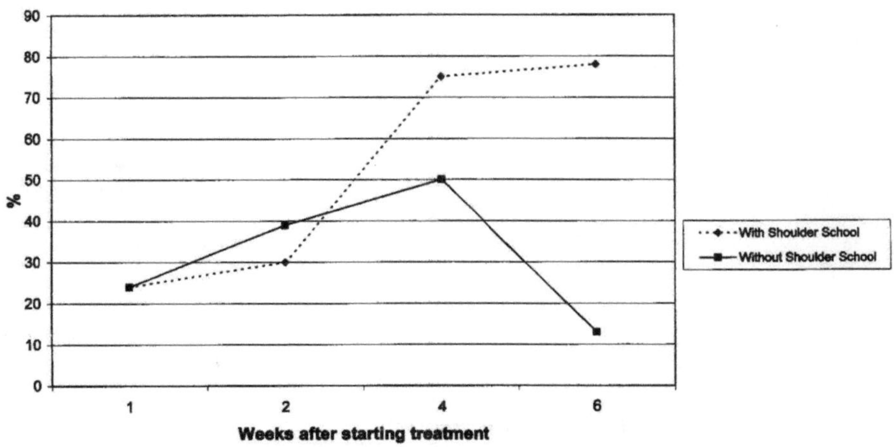

Fig. 1. Explained variance of muscular strength in shoulder patients due to health locus of control

arm such as internal rotation and external rotation in adduction); mobility of the shoulder joint in flexion, abduction, adduction as well as internal rotation and external rotation in adduction. The health locus of control became measured at the time of the first examination by the GKÜ-scale (Böhlen 1987; see also Nentwig and Windemuth 1993). This scale measures the health-locus of control on the dimensions internality (e.g. "diseases of many people are the result of their own carelessness"); p-externality (e.g. "the treatment of diseases belongs in the hands of a specialist"); and c-externality (e.g. "my health depends mainly on fate"). Patients had to specify their agreement on a rating scale between the extremes 1 (exactly right) and 6 (not correct at all).

For knee patients the convalescence was evaluated by the criteria of muscular strength based on the girth of the leg 10 and 20 cm above the knee, different pain measures and the degree of mobility of the knee joint. Out of this measure three indices were computed: for muscular strength, for pain and for mobility. All measures were taken 1, 2, 4 and 8 weeks after the start of treatment (Fig. 2). The psychological variables are measured in the same way as for the shoulder patients.

The results of the correlation analyses between patients with and without shoulder and knee school are particularly interesting (Figs. 1 and 2). The criterion of *muscular strength* can be observed: 1 week after the first examination 24% of the variance within both groups of shoulder patients can be explained by the results of locus of control (Fig. 1). In the second week, 30% of the variance can be explained for patients with shoulder school and 39% for the patients without this training. In the fourth and eighth weeks there were different trends: while for patients without

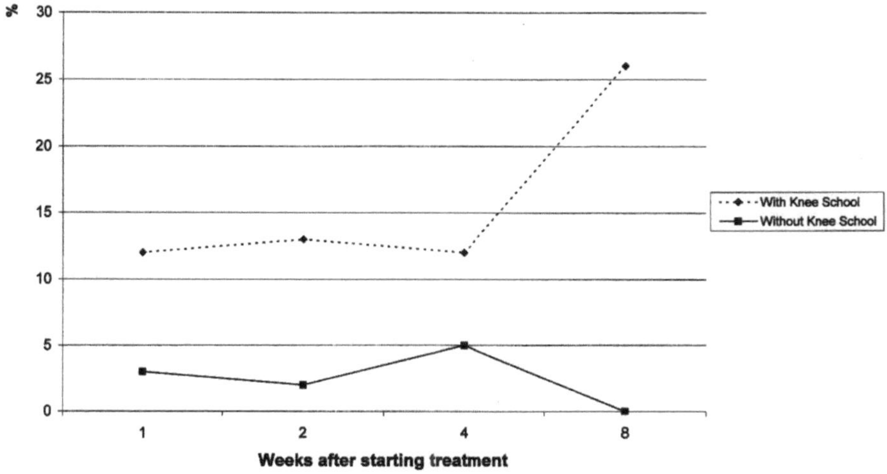

Fig. 2. Explained variance of muscular strength in knee patients due to health locus of control

shoulder school there was an increase to 50% in the fourth week, and after this a decrease to only 13% after 8 weeks, those with shoulder school showed the percentage of explained variance increases to a high level with 75% in the fourth and 78% in the eighth week after start of the treatment.

The course for the knee patients was a little different. While for patients without knee school there was no prediction of muscular strength due to locus of control there was an increasing explanation of variance from the fourth to the sixth week from 12% to 26% for patients with knee school.

All in all, the variance of muscular strength after beginning medical therapy or medical therapy combined with behavioral training can be explained due to health locus of control for patients trained to behave in the right way to increase their muscular strength. Locus of control is unimportant for patients not receiving information about the possibilities of training.

A look at the explanation of the variance of pain intensity can prove this hypothesis that health locus of control is an important variable for convalescence, but that it is of importance only if the patients learns what to do during convalescence. Because no patients in the study learned about pain control, this variance should not be explainable. In fact there was no significant influence on this variance due to locus of control (always less than 1.5%).

In the context of training therapy these results are a large source of expression of the importance of health locus of control. They prove that locus of control predicts the practice of specific behavior, e.g. physical training for muscular strengthening. For variables such as pain, on which no possibilities of influence were obtained, it does not have importance. Since training therapy always implies independent behavior of the participants, as a determinant of this behavior locus of control is obviously of great importance.

Study II: Replication of Results from Study I for Surgical Patients after Rupture of a Ligament of the Knee Joint

The second study was performed in $n=95$ patients after surgery of the anterior cruciate ligament or medial collateral ligament. These injuries are rarely seen solely (see Karpf and Mang 1981). That is why patients with additional damage of the meniscii etc. were included. After an initial 2-week stationary treatment (surgery, thigh plaster cast, first gymnastic exercises) patients were dismissed from the hospital for approximately 4 weeks. During this time patients should continue the exercise by themselves (e.g. static contraction exercises). Subsequently, they were taken up a second time for 2 weeks (plaster cast removal and physical exercises). Convalescence could be diagnosed and quantified at the beginning and at the end of the second treatment phase: the muscle atrophy in the thigh at 10 and 20 cm above the knee, knee joint swelling, and exact range of the knee in relation to the untreated leg. The mobility of the knee joint could be measured in degrees. Additionally, in a partially structured interview the well-being of the patients was assessed. The GKÜ-questionnaire was given 2–3 days after the surgery. This is the first study specifically showing that the phase outside the clinic provides the opportunity for the patients to influence convalescence by independent exercises.

The key question is: can the independent behavior be predicted by health locus of control? This is of importance for the success of training programs such as knee, shoulder or back schools. This behavior, and thus, convalescence should be predictable by the health locus of control.

For the purpose of the evaluation patients were divided into two groups according to the medical diagnosis (a value combined from the different criteria). The first group is called "well convalescence", the second group "bad convalescence". The criterion "well" or "bad" is determined over the average value of the total group. Those with worse diagnostic values than the total group average are classified as "bad convalescence". Those who obtain better values are classified as "well convalescence". With the help of comprehensive statistical procedures, we can now see whether this allocation to one of the two groups is predictable from the psychological status. The result of this statistical analysis is shown in Table 1. For nearly 72% of the patients, due to their health locus of control, the group to which they will belong 6 weeks after surgery can be predicted. The patients with an unfavorable convalescence believe significantly more in the importance of medical personnel for their health (p-externality). In view of the fact that no prediction is possible from medical variables, the computed percentage is amazingly high. On the basis of chance a hit rate of approximately 50% would be expected.

Table 1. Results of the statistical analysis when patients were divided into good and bad convalescence

	Good convalescence	Bad convalescence
Actual diagnosis	32.1%	39.6%
Incorrect diagnosis	13.2%	15.1%

Percentage of correctly classified patients: 71.7%; for 32.1% the prognosis "good convalescence" was correct, while for 39.6% the prognosis "bad convalescence" was correct. For 13.2% and 15.1%, respectively, an incorrect prognosis was obtained.

The attempt to identify patients who benefited from independent exercises on the basis of psychological characteristics was successful to a large extent. Patients believing medical personnel as unimportant for their health status benefit mostly from the phase of independent exercises. Patients believing medical personnel as important do not benefit from the period of independent exercises.

Consequences for Practice

What are the consequences for practice that can be derived from this result? Wallston and Wallston (1978) discuss changing the locus of control beliefs with patients in order to develop a favorable behavior. However, they present the possibility of using health locus of control as an indication variable in order to tailor therapy to each patient.

Changing Health Locus of Control to Increase the Success of Training Therapy

With the justified assumption that control beliefs (mediated, e.g. by the regularity of gymnastic exercises) have an influence on the health and convalescence of patients, the question about a change of these beliefs is of great practical importance. Can patients achieve an increase of compliance by internalization? Nearly all studies on the connection between control beliefs and health are correlational under the assumption of mediating variables; however, a causal connection can be made plausible. The extent of the compliance is determined by the control beliefs and thus the quality of convalescence is also controlled by these beliefs.

Studies with the aim of increasing global internality originate predominantly from the 1970s. To reach this goal programs of information transfer and more practically aligned procedures are conceivable (MacDonald 1972). An overview of the few attempts to change locus of control can be found in Wallston et al. (1978) and also Krampen (1982, 1985). Furthermore, Krampen identifies fundamental methodological weaknesses of most of these studies such as different evaluation criteria, no accurate description of the therapeutic procedure, exclusive view of a possible internalization. Overall most studies seem to be promising, whereby increasing internality seems to be successful following programs for modification of behavior or if reinforcements are contingent to a behavior; examples are: training for the increase of social competence (Dua 1970) programs for modification of health behavior (weight reduction: Tobias and MacDonald 1977), stationary psychotherapy (without specification: Gillis and Jessor 1970), interventions for the management of an acute life crisis (Smith 1970) or by token or particularly aligned relaxation programs with systematic employment of social reinforcements with children (Nowicki and Barnes 1973; Gutkin 1978).

Diamond and Shapiro (1973) discuss the possibility that if therapy or an intervention serves as a behavioral model, then internalization of the participant would be a consequence of modeling. Discussion, suggestion or meditation as interventions, in which reinforcements of learned new behavior will be experienced only slightly are suitable as planned relaxation programs but not particularly for the modification of control beliefs (Dua 1970; Page 1975; Zuroff and Schwarz 1978). In no study was the change of the control beliefs assessed on a long-term basis. Considerations of Lau (1982) that locus of control can be changed with difficulty do not contradict the empirical results. Lau (1982) summarizes efforts toward a change of the health locus of control referring to Wallston et al. (1981) and Lefcourt (1976) in the following way: "None of these experiments were successful in changing HLC [Health Locus of Control] beliefs, although all were designed to do just that ..." (p 332). At least the global locus of control is easier to change than the health-specific one.

Altogether, it is to be noted that a change of health-specific control beliefs can be meaningful for the increase of the effect of the training therapy. So far there has been no description of an effective way to change these area-specific beliefs. Thus, another possibility must be found in order to make the research results usable in practice.

Using Health Locus of Control as an Indication Variable

More effective and less complex than the modification of control beliefs is the tailoring of treatment to the patient's locus of control. Krampen (1982) outlined in the framework of psychotherapy, two different kinds of indication. Locus of control is important both in a selective indication model, according to which patients are suitable for a certain psychotherapy, and in an adaptive indication model (Zielke 1979), according to which an optimal adjustment of the therapeutic procedure to the characteristics of the client are aimed (p 177).

Adaptive indication models due to locus of control of patients worked with different forms of the psychotherapy (e.g. Kilmann et al. 1975; Best 1975; Best and Steffy 1975). For internal clients, those interventions that are less structured seem to be effective. For external clients, more structured and more organized therapies are effective.

In the area of medical treatment with and without additional behavior modification, such studies are rare. For instance, Wiltse and Rocchio (1975) provide a selective indication for disc operations due to the scale profiles in the MMPI. Due to the control beliefs, no indication models have been set up so far. This is particularly notable, since locus of control has been proved to be a health-relevant variable, e.g. for the behavior that is important for the success of a training therapy. The establishment of an indication variable like locus of control would cause an increase in the effectiveness of the treatment. However, treatment success can also be increased with patients who do not profit from behavior training programs; for such patients more favorable treatment forms are made available. The past studies for the usability of the control beliefs as an indication variable are not sufficient however, in order to create a general indication model. In the context of medical treatment, as in the context of psychological supply, a high degree of responsibility is suggested to be given to internal patients. For p-external patients, controlled treatment seems to be more effective. If such a indication model is developed, this not only increases the effectiveness of many treatments; at the same time substantial costs could be saved in the health service, because individually ineffective treatments would less frequently be prescribed.

References

Best JA (1975) Tailoring smoking withdrawal procedures to personality and motivational differences. J Consult Clin Psychol 43:1–8

Best JA, Steffy, RA (1975) Smoking modification procedures for internal and external locus of control clients. Can J Behavioural Science 7:155–165

Böhlen G (1987) Kontrollüberzeugung und Gesundheit. Entwicklung einer Skala und Untersuchungen zur "Sozialen Erwünschtheit". Unveröff. Examensarbeit, Universität Duisburg, Duisburg

Calsyn DA, Louks J, Freeman CW (1976) The use of the MMPI with chronic low back pain patients with a mixed diagnosis. J Clin Psychol 32:532–536

Constant CR, Murley AHG (1987) A clinical method of functional assessment of the shoulder. Clin Orthop 214:160–164

Diamond J, Shapiro JL (1973) Changes in locus of control as a function of encounter group experience: a study and replication. J Abnorm Psychol 82:514–518

Dua PS (1970) Comparison of the effect of behaviorally oriented action and psychotherapy reeducation on introversion-extraversion, emotionality, and internal-external control. J Consult Clin Psychol 17:567–572

Ferring D, Filipp S-H (1989) Der Fragebogen zur Erfassung gesundheitsbezogener Kontrollüberzeugungen (FEGK). Z Klein Psychologie 18:285–289

Gillis JS, Jessor L (1970) Effects of brief psychotherapy on belief in internal control: an exploratory study. Psychotherapy 7:135–137

Grifka J (1992) Die Knieschule. Rowohlt, Reinbek

Gutkin TB (1978) Modification of elementary students' locus of control: an operant approach. J Psychol 100:107–115

Hanvik LJ (1951) MMPI problems in patients with low-back pain. J Consult Clin Psychol 15:350–353

Hasenbrink M, Ahrens S (1987) Depressivität, Schmerzwahrnehmung und Schmerzerleben bei Patienten mit lumbalem Bandscheibenvorfall. Psychotherapie, Psychosomatik und Medizinische Psychologie 37:149–155

Hedtmann A, Fett H (1988) Schulterschule. Orthopädische Praxis, Sonderausgabe zur 36. Jahrestagung der Vereinigung Süddeutscher Orthopäden pp 76–77

Hirsch C (1965) Efficiency of surgery in low-back-disorders. Pathoanatomical, experimental, and clinical studies. J Bone Joint Surg 47A:991–1004
Karpf PM, Mang W (1981) Diagnostisches Vorgehen bei frischen Knieinnenverletzungen. In: D Hohmann (ed) Praktische Orthopädie, Band 11: Das Knie (Hrsg. E. Rausch). Stork, Bruchsal, pp 399–404
Kilmann PR, Albert BM, Sotile WM (1975) Relationship between locus of control, structure of therapy, and outcome. J Consult Clin Psychol 43:588
Kohlmann CW, Küstner E, Beyer J (1993) Kontrollüberzeugungen und Diabeteseinstellung in Abhängigkeit von der Art der Erkrankungsdauer. Z Gesundheitspsychologie 1:32–48
Krampen G (1982) Differentialpsychologie der Kontrollüberzeugungen ("Locus of Control"). Hogrefe, Göttingen
Krampen G (1985) Zur Bedeutung von Kontrollüberzeugungen in der klinischen Psychologie. Z Klin Psychologie 14:101–112
Lau RR (1982) Origins of health locus of control beliefs. J Pers Social Psychol 42:322–334
Lefcourt HM (1976) Locus of control: current trends in theory and research. Erlbaum, Hillsdale
Levenson H (1972) Activism and powerful others: distinction within the concept of internal-external control. J Pers Assess 38:237–383
Lohaus A, Schmitt M (1988) Fragebogen zur Erhebung von Kontrollüberzeugungen zu Krankheit und Gesundheit (KKG). Hogrefe, Göttingen
MacDonald AP (1972) Internal-external locus of control change-techniques. Rehab Lit 33:44–47
Merskey H, Boyd D (1978) Emotional adjustment and chronic pain. Pain 5:173–178
Mrazek J (1989) Die Erfassung körperbezogener Kontrollüberzeugungen. In: G Krampen (ed) Diagnostik von Attributionen und Kontrollüberzeugungen. Hogrefe, Göttingen, pp 112–118
Neer CS II (1983) Impingement lesions. Clin Orthop 173:70–77
Nentwig CG, Krämer J, Ullrich CH (1990) Die Rückenschule. Enke, Stuttgart
Nentwig CG, Windemuth D (1992) Entwicklung und Validierung einer kurzen Skala zur Erfassung des Verstärkungswertes der Gesundheit. Verhaltensmodifikation und Verhaltensmedizin 13:217–234
Nowicki S, Barnes J (1973) Effects of a structured camp experience on locus of control orientation. J Gen Psychol 122:247–252
Oostdam EMM, Duivenvoorden HJ (1983) Predictability of the result of surgical intervention in patients with low back pain. J Psychosom Res 27:273–281
Page WF (1975) Self-esteem and internal versus external control among black youth in a summer aviation program. J Psychol 89:307–311
Partridge C, Johnston M (1989) Perceived control of recovery from physical disability: measurement and prediction. Br J Clin Psychol 28:53–59
Roberts N, Smith R, Bennett S, Cape J (1984) Health beliefs and rehabilitation after lumbar disc surgery. J Psychosom Res 28:139–144
Rogner O, Frey D, Havemann D (1987) Der Genesungsverlauf von Unfallpatienten aus kognitions-psychologischer Sicht. Z Klinische Psychologie 16:11–28
Rotter JB (1954) Social learning and clinical psychology. Prentice-Hall, New York
Rotter JB (1966) Generalized expectancies for internal versus external control of reinforcement. Psychological Monographs 80 (1, whole No. 609)
Rotter JB (1975) Some problems and misconceptions related to the construct of internal vs. external control of reinforcement. J Consult Clin Psychol 43:56–67
Schulze C, Florin I, Matschin E, Sougioultzi C, Schulze HH (1988) Psychological distress after hysterectomy – a predictive study. Psychol Health 2:1–12

Schumacher M, Ehlers A, Ulshöfer B (1987) Einfluß medizinischer, psychologischer und sozialer Variablen auf den Rehabilitationsverlauf Nierensteinerkrankter nach extrakorporaler Nierensteinzertrümmerung (ESWL). Referat auf dem 1. Kongreß der Deutschen Gesellschaft für Verhaltensmedizin und Verhaltensmodifikation in München

Schwetschenau PR, Ramirez A, Johnston J, Barnes E, Wiggs C, Martins AN (1976) Double-blind evaluation of intradiscal chymopapain for herniated lumbar discs. J Neurosurg 45:622–627

Smith RE (1970) Changes in locus of control as a function of life crises resolution. J Abnorm Psychol 75:328–332

Sternbach RA, Wolf SR, Murphy RW, Akeson WH (1973) Traits of pain patients: the low-back "loser". Psychosomatics 14:226–229

Tobias LT, MacDonald M (1977) Internal locus of control and weight loss: an insufficient condition. J Consult Clin Psychol 45:647–653

Valach L, Augustiny KF, Dvorak J, Blaser P, Fuhrimann P, Tschaggelar W, Heim E (1988) Coping von rückenoperierten Patienten - psychosoziale Aspekte. Psychotherapie, Psychosomatik und Medizinische Psychologie 38:28–36

Wallston BS, Wallston KA (1978) Locus of control and health: a review of the literature. Health Education Monographs 6:107–117

Wallston KA, Wallston BS (1981) Health locus of control. In: HM Lefcourt (ed) Research with the locus of control construct 1. Academic Press, New York, pp 189–243

Wallston KA, Wallston BS, Kaplan GD, Maides SA (1976) Development and validation of the health locus of control (HLC) scale. J Consult Clin Psychol 44:580–585

Wallston KA, Wallston BS, DeVellis R (1978) Development of the multidimensional health locus of control (MHLC) scales. Health Education Monographs 6:160–170

Waring EM, Weisz GM, Bailey I (1976) Predictive factors in the treatment of low back pain by surgical intervention. Adv Pain Res Therapy 1:939–942

Weir BKA (1979) Prospective study of 100 lumbo-sacral discectomies. J Neurosurg 50:283–289

World Health Organization (1986) Ottawa charter for health promotion. WHO, Geneva

Wiltse LL, Rocchio PD (1975) Preoperative psychological tests as predictors of success of chemonucleolysis in the treatment of the low-back syndrome. J Bone Joint Surg 57:478–483

Windemuth D (1991) Die Vorhersage der Gesundung von Patienten durch gesundheitsbezogene Kontrollüberzeugungen. Kovac, Hamburg

Windemuth D, Nentwig CG, Böhlen G, Hierholzer G (1991) Vorhersage der organischen Rekonvaleszenz durch gesundheitsspezifische Kontrollüberzeugungen nach Kniegelenkbandoperationen. Z Klinische Psychologie 20:128–135

Windemuth D, Ullrich CH (1997) Knie- und Schulterschulen. In: CG Nentwig, J Krämer, CH Ullrich (eds) Die Rückenschule. 3. Auflage, Enke, Stuttgart, pp 77–81

Zielke M (1979) Indikation zur Gesprächspsychotherapie. Kohlhammer, Stuttgart

Zuroff DC, Schwarz JC (1978) Effects of transcendental meditation and muscle relaxation on trait anxiety, maladjustment, locus of control, and drug use. J Consult Clin Psychol 46:264–271

Subject Index

O

P

R

S

MIX
Papier aus verantwortungsvollen Quellen
Paper from responsible sources
FSC® C105338

If you have any concerns about our products,
you can contact us on
ProductSafety@springernature.com

In case Publisher is established outside the EU,
the EU authorized representative is:
Springer Nature Customer Service Center GmbH
Europaplatz 3, 69115 Heidelberg, Germany

Printed by Libri Plureos GmbH
in Hamburg, Germany